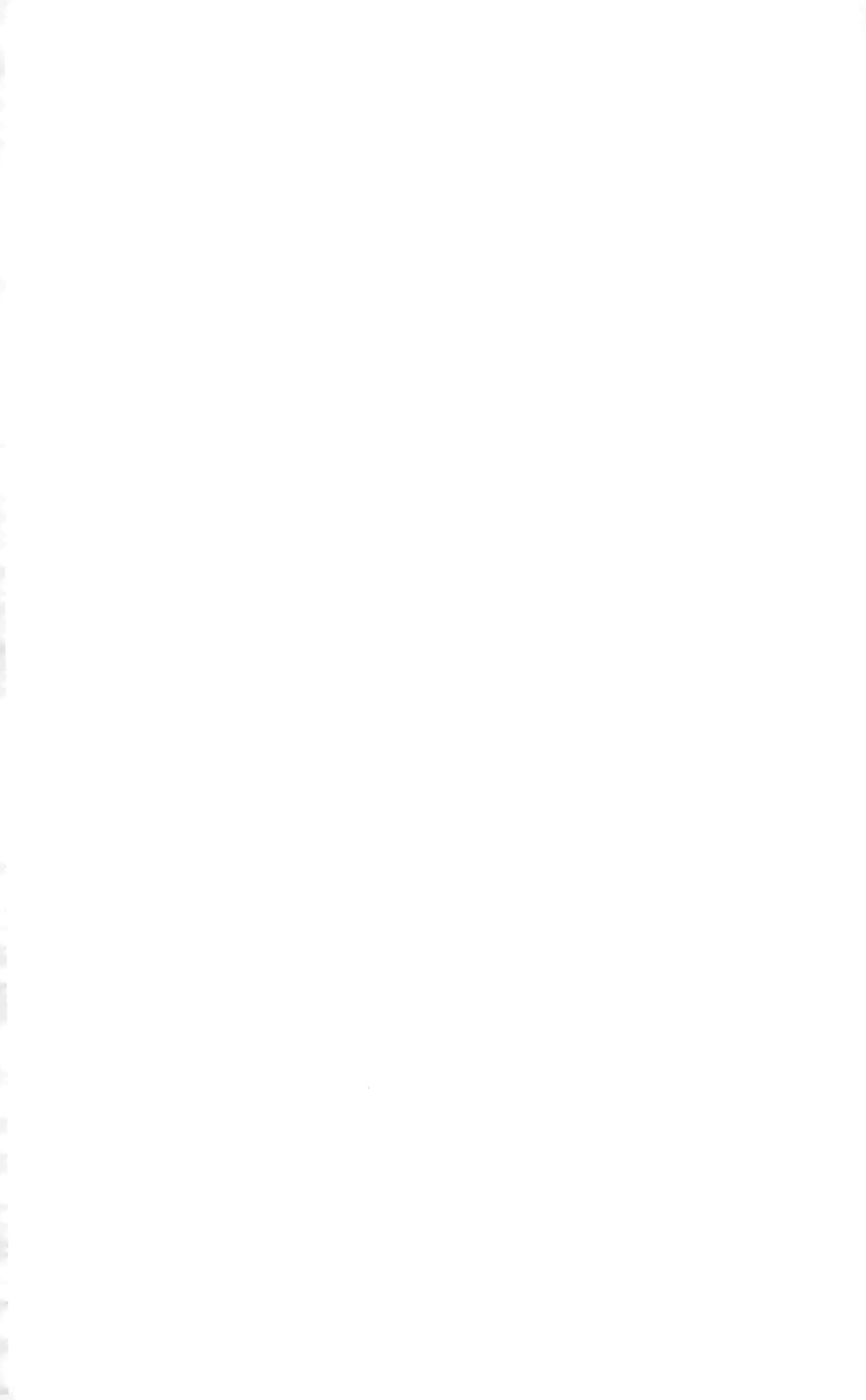

Printed in Victoria, Canada

**Canadian Cataloguing in Publication Data**

Lesser, Gershon M.
Healing and spirit

ISBN 1-55212-394-4

1. Lesser, Gershon M. 2. Physicians--United States --Biography. I. Harding, Mitchell II. Title.
R154.L45A3 2000 610'.92 C00-910868-8

TRAFFORD

**This book was published *on-demand* in cooperation with Trafford Publishing.**
On-demand publishing is a unique process and service of making a book available for retail sale to the public taking advantage of on-demand manufacturing and Internet marketing. **On-demand publishing** includes promotions, retail sales, manufacturing, order fulfilment, accounting and collecting royalties on behalf of the author.

Suite 6E, 2333 Government St., Victoria, B.C. V8T 4P4, CANADA
Phone 250-383-6864 Toll-free 1-888-232-4444 (Canada & US)
Fax 250-383-6804 E-mail sales@trafford.com
Web site www.trafford.com TRAFFORD PUBLISHING IS A DIVISION OF TRAFFORD HOLDINGS LTD.
Trafford Catalogue #00-0058 www.trafford.com/robots/00-0058.html

10 9 8 7 6 5 4 3 2

# Healing and Spirit

## Medicine, Politics, Civilization And The Making Of An Extraordinary Physician

*Gershon Lesser, MD*

*&*

*Mitchell Harding*

Trafford Publishing

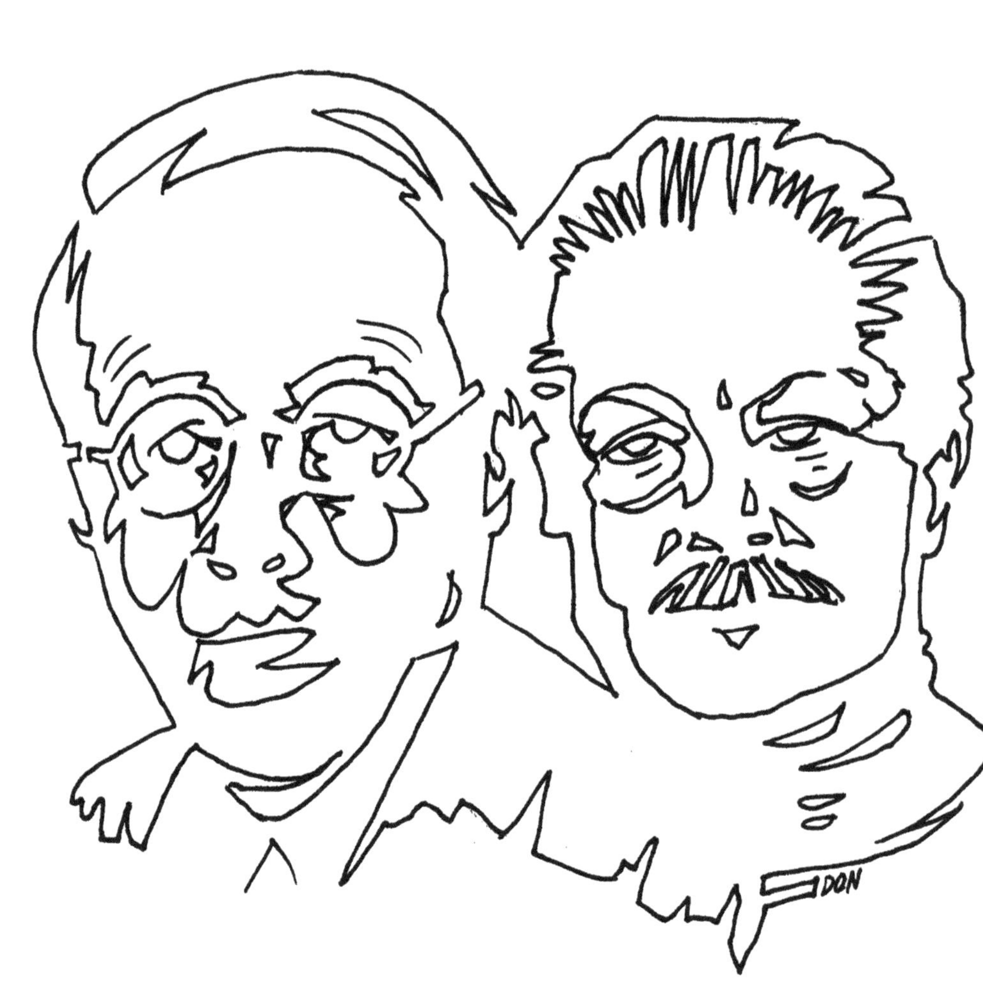
DON

***"We heal each other not because we are sick,
but because we are holy."***

# CONTENTS

# INTRODUCTION

You are about to meet an extraordinary man, a physician with 40 years of medical experience, who can no longer bear to witness the spiritual crisis of modern medicine and the malaise of America, without crying out. This is the inspired and rational doctor we all want today and cannot find.

Physicians such as Dr. Lesser know that we are more than just collections of secretions and tubing. His primary mission is to awaken you to heal yourself. He is concerned with the ignition of thought and the launching of your inner power. He is concerned with your fear, joy, moral bedrock, and the gentle mix of compromises which can make life worth living. This book is about your mind and soul as much as your health.

Health lies in your awareness, your consciousness, your willingness to recognize the malignant essences of fear and anger. People sense there is more to life and health than pills and, everywhere they are seeking transcendence and completion. Dr. Lesser can help you in your search. When you finish this book, you will know whether you need to go pill hunting or not.

Some of the chapters below are devoted to introducing Dr. Lesser. Before he can convincingly express his intense indignation at the state of modern medicine, and other harmful forces destroying your health, and your country, you must know who he is, and that he can be trusted. We must be grounded in bedrock before we can follow him to the fall of empires.

There are chapters ahead on AIDS and cancer, picking your doctor and alternative medicine, ecology and God, television and sex. This is not a pill book; it's a book about healing. The good doctor saves his finest invective and highest dudgeon for the chapter on HMO's, which is thrown into high relief by a reprint of the original Oath of Hippocrates, also included, still sworn by many doctors today.

I should also mention the three amusing Lesser Arcana "dramatic" productions, the many stories from Dr. Lesser's medical career, and an extraordinary and terrifying "dark night of the soul" which I (MH) feel has not been equaled since St. John of the Cross wrote in the 16th. century!

Your mental and spiritual health is the underlying theme of this book. From the privacy of your soul, to the thousand year tides of history, here is a magnificent survey, on the largest scale, of *what medicine, civilization and religion should be*, and too often are not. You should keep this book at hand as an introduction to the biggest picture if you must take your pills

A word or two about the other writer of *Healing and Spirit.* Born Eugene Loring Ware, I come from an old American WASP family, lower middle class, middle 1930's, middle brow, out of the Steppes of Central Illinois (Urbana). I am retired from a 35 year career in non-commercial radio under the name Mitchell Harding.

You will know me from a list of my heroes. In no particular order they are Buckminster Fuller, Edward James Olmos, Frederick Douglass, Lorenzo di Medici, Jean-Pierre Hallet, the ancient Greeks, Studs Terkel, Julia Hill, Paul Robeson, Elie Wiesel, Malcolm X, Black Elk, I.F. Stone, Osaka, The Dalai Lama, Thomas Jefferson, and Jim Hensen; all warriors of the mind and spirit; all speakers of truth, pleasant or not.

Gershon is a fine writer in his own right. He has a poetic, and marvelously complex mind. What is my role in this book? I am the disentangler, straightener, expander, and clarifier, but I have tried to keep the good doctor's essence intact in whatever I touched.

I need to thank my brother Don Ware, the talented one in the family, for the light hearted interior illustrations. I must also express my thanks to my brother and to my son, Julian Ross Ware, for their insightful and necessary criticisms and corrections. Some of it was hard to take. Thanks to Stan Brumer for telling us what we needed to know, and for some essential boiler plate, and Alan Ogden for rescuing our book from a Black Hole it had fallen into. OK, Gershon. It's all yours.

- Mitchell Harding

Thanks Mitch.

I must thank Dr. Jerome S. Tamkin, Judith Tamkin, and the Tamkin Foundation for invaluable inspiration and support all along the way. Thanks to Irvin Atkins, producer of my program series on KGIL, National Public Radio station KCRW for 18 years of hospitality to what I had to say, and the Los Angeles County Medical Association for my stint as host of their television program Healthline

- Dr. Gershon Lesser

This morning I was having breakfast with my wife and looking through the newspaper. I suddenly realized my heart rate was increasing. I don't have to take my pulse any more with this noisy mechanical heart valve. I'm wondering why am I getting anxious when I'm having a simple breakfast with a pleasant person beside me.

Then I realized that everything I was reading was of moral bankruptcy. A corporation was laying off 40,000 people, some of whom had been there 18 years, losing their retirement and health benefits. I read of a 14 year old girl who was shot in the head in a random drive-by shooting. I read of the two children of a University of Southern California (USC) faculty member who died of a heroin overdose, and of the well known popular singer who was acquitted of a murder he had admitted to reporters. There was the usual "news" of riot and mayhem, of pain and suffering, of starvation and corruption, of hypocrisy and scorn for our fellow human beings. Nowhere was there any evidence of love. A newspaper for breakfast was just as devastating to my health as the fried eggs and sausage on my plate.

In a world encased in pain and suffering, I offer you my outstretched hands. The door is open. Your humanity, dear friend, has been ignored. You have been disenfranchised; by your lawyer, your boss, your politicians, your mate, your children, your society, your doctor; and all the list making, bean counting, lint picking, instant health touted by the thousands of "self help" books in your book stores. They have their place. I wrote a marvelous one myself recently, but we need more than that.

All of us need healing, and we need to talk.

# 1

## Heart Failure

*"Welcome to Doctor Gershon Lesser's Health Connection. Dr. Lesser is an internist and cardiologist, and a founding member of the International Academy of Preventive Medicine. Also an attorney, he has received White House honors for his efforts in bringing preventive medicine to the public. And now, Doctor Gershon Lesser."*

Every Wednesday afternoon for 18 years the announcer introduced my call-in programs on National Public Radio with those old familiar words. I have also had scheduled programs on nine commercial radio stations and ten television stations in Southern California, New Mexico, Hawaii, and Alaska, as well as Canada and South Africa. My programs have been carried from time to time on network radio and television and national cable, as well as being picked up occasionally by hundreds of other radio and television stations around the country. It's possible you may have heard my voice. I've answered a lot of your telephone calls. I know how much health interests you.

What I am about to tell you may echo your own medical experiences. All of us have medical stories that we wish weren't true. I had been a doctor for over 30 years. I fully intended to die in my boots at age 130, practicing internal medicine and doing my weekly radio program. But life is not a sitcom and even doctors sometimes encounter reality. The bottom dropped out of my life and I became a patient.

My aortic valve replacement was not exactly a surprise. The alleged reason I went into heart surgery was a sudden discovery of a congenital defect in the aortic valve that had overgrown with calcium. I was over the age of 50. I was a smoker for years. Almost every heart patient is. I was overweight. I was a workaholic. I was depressed. I really didn't take care of myself the way I had asked others to do for themselves. I didn't tell the truth to myself. None of us do. In my early years I had participated in physical fitness programs and yoga but recently I had given up exercise.

This is all mixed up in my mind with the death of my son. I haven't yet discovered how to express my rage. I'm not quite sure how far to go in expressing it here. It runs from my guilt at not keeping him home, to the threat from his professor to lower his A+ grade if he didn't go on the trip, to the indifference of his school after he died. He was one of two killed in the accident, and I have no answers.

Wasn't I in fact very much a high risk patient who didn't need the excuse of a congenitally deformed valve? You won't be surprised to know that I wasn't "*mature, disinterested, and professional*" in what follows.

Here is what it really felt like! Having walked up to the hospital's main entrance, I was forced into a wheelchair and rolled into the hospital. With my heart leaping in my chest, I ended up first in the hospital insurance office. "*When people come in, the first thing we have to do is business,*" the receptionist reminded me. From that moment on no one cared to do anything with my life but stay in control of it for their own convenience. This sounds familiar to you doesn't it, dear friend, but it was new to me.

Upstairs I put on that offensive gown. Sometime I may do a paper on The Psychology of Leaving Our Luscious Buns Bare In Public. I arranged for an expensive private room so that my wife could sleep there, but it was too small to open her bed. She had to sleep on a hardback chair.

The very fine famous surgeon who was going to operate on me told me I had an aortic stenosis. "*It's significant, and it needs to be replaced with a mechanical valve. You have no choice if you want to live*," he said. As I remember that day today in tranquillity, I think he was wrong!

My surgery would occur at 6:30 AM the following morning. That night I was served a choice of wine, lobster, steak, all the things you don't serve a cardiac patient unless you don't expect them to live through it. Tests were arranged.

I was terror stricken. The very fine technicians had to get the computers to the right temperature, have a cup of coffee, and joke with each other over my pale, sweating, overweight, middle aged, terrified, naked body. There was no one to reassure me, no one to figuratively hold my hand during the multiple invasive procedures. I was discovering things, as a patient, that most of you have known all along about hospitals and medicine.

I was moved to a smaller room. I had been pre-empted by a very fine Mideastern millionaire and his extended family.

My mind was in a whirl at 6:30 AM. I was given sedatives, that didn't work very well, to take away my fear that I would die. I thought that it would be worth while if I could trade places with my dead son and give him his life back. Just for a moment, in a sudden strange guilt, I had the thought that perhaps he had traded his life for mine. I wanted to be able to speak to somebody.

The doctors were no help. There is no one in our world who can help us through a spiritual crisis like this except the dedicated divines attached to the churches and synagogues. I use the word dedicated in two senses. All of us discover that we must sign up and register in a particular creed and set of practices before we can be talked to by an accredited certified representative of God. This is not the function of psychology. What shrink or advisor will take on this responsibility? Our loved ones are not ready for this great charge. *Who ministers to humanity?*

After I was asleep, marvelous people were going to put me on a table and strip me down, the way a dead body might be prepared. Even a physician can feel deep in his soul that they are planning to chop open his chest with a hatchet. There was still no one to talk to about any of this.

A cheery anesthesiologist came by who cheerily said good morning and cheerily started me into sedation. Then I was operated on, but I wasn't there.

❄

For at least an hour or three, or 24, after the operation, I was totally unaware. There was an intravenous tube (IV) in each arm, and wires sticking out all over the place, and I didn't have any idea who I was, where I was, or what was happening. It would have been nice to have someone sitting there to welcome me back to the world.

There were timeless moments when I didn't have any reaction at all, until I finally became quite frantic. I focused on the basics. I'm Gershon Lesser. I am a patient. I just had heart surgery. I have a wife and two sons. I just lost a third son. I live where, and with whom? Why? What now?

I began my search for meaning. My judgment wandered in pathways of which I couldn't make sense.

There is a world literature of illumination and epiphany coming out of the worst possible circumstances. Would we Americans be better off if we were trained to serenity, mindfulness, acceptance, transcendence, and the yoga of the moment, no matter what it was, before being confronted with our mortality by some surgeon in a shining white operating room? After an operation do we experience with our liver, our heart, or our mind?

Recovering in my new room, I was shocked awake by loud rock music, an early morning favorite of one of the marvelous millionaire's extended family. The operative word was panic - continuous shocking panic! I was clutching a hornet's nest to my chest!

I asked for a special cardiac nurse to stay with me at night because I was still fearful of all the things that could go wrong. Being a physician I was triply fearful because I understood things that patients don't ordinarily perceive. He said, "*Yes I'll stay if you're willing to pay my fee of 1,000 dollars.*" I told him okay. He never showed up.

In my third day in the hospital, completely bedridden, with a catheter up my penis, I was being bathed buck naked by a very fine young nurse, the water cold, her mind elsewhere. She told me her financial problems, how tough life was for her, and I had to listen. Panic!

She rolled me over onto one side, totally unaware that the catheter was pinned down to the sheet. I yelled, "*Oh my God,*

*You're castrating me!*" "*Oh yeah, it's pinned down,*" was her only comment. Surely any trained nurse, or even someone with a normal amount of human empathy, would have known to unpin catheters and other wires and tubes before moving someone who was just out of major surgery. A human being would have taken more care to unplug a toaster before moving it. A human being would have apologized. Today I have a new perception of the nursing profession.

They sent up an intern, a very fine young man, who became annoyed at my complaints. They had made him run upstairs to visit me. He assured me that my EKG was perfectly normal, and I pointed out that it wasn't perfectly normal 30 minutes ago, when I buzzed the nurse. No one was sympathetic. Now I was getting angry. I guess I was recovering.

The next morning, another marvelous intern announced that he was going to remove two huge drains that were in my chest wall. I asked, "*Where was the surgeon?*" I was told that surgeons of that stature don't remove drains. He assured me he had done 21 and was now an expert. I was supposed to be calm and stay in my place. I was worried, but he performed the procedure.

The fine nurse gruffly had me walk barefoot to the bathroom. When I pointed out that no one had put any slippers out, she told me I wouldn't need them anyway, it was a clean floor. "*Come on,*" I said, trying to reason with her. "*You're worried about me becoming infected with hospital bacteria. That's why you're bathing me so much. But I haven't seen anyone come into this room to clean the toilet, or sterilize the floor since I arrived. I'm a physician, and I know that hospital infections are all over. Where is your janitor?*"

A very professional woman came in to give me an injection, then turned around and left when she realized the injection was for someone else. Food trays were often left across the room, or on the table near my bed, but not close enough for me to reach them or eat from them. If someone in my family didn't walk in I wouldn't have been able to eat.

**We would all probably go stark staring mad if it ever occurred to us that every single person we will ever see is a human being just like us!**

Where do I put my anger? I felt no sacred bliss in being alive, in being empowered to give birth to myself. I was ill. I was sad. During the operation my heart was stopped, and the blood supply to my brain had been interrupted. No one reminded me that would happen. I grasped my anguish! The harder and harder I held it, the hotter and hotter the sting of it became. I was addicted to it. I couldn't let go! I did the opposite of what I am trying to teach here! As I write I am finally beginning to see my need to give up my anger. Yet I'm still angry, and I have so far to go.

Surgery is cutting. No matter how shining the knives, how careful the anesthesia, how well trained the butchers, we are being sorely wounded under the surgeon's scalpel. It does not occur to us that surgery is a knife assault, no different to the body's healing mechanisms than something done to us with a switchblade in a dark alley. The shining chromium tools and fixtures hide a medieval, and even sometimes barbaric, core.

Since the days of the Roman Empire the prime precept of medical ethics has always been, "*Primum Non Nocere*" (above all, do no harm). Think twice before you opt for surgery. I suppose it is too much to ask that doctors see this more clearly, but I don't think it is too much to ask that they discover humility more often! I can't put down my rage at the failure of the surgeons to have addressed the issues fully with me before the operation, discussed it and placed it all on the balance. I am not a number!

Personal contact down - malpractice suits up! I am beginning to understand why this can be. According to one study, there seems to be an inverse correlation between the time a physician spends with his or her patient and the number of malpractice suits filed. My surgeon knew nothing of me or my confusion.

I'm still caught up in all the turmoil of having a heart operation, of a later bladder hemorrhage, of being forced to conclude my practice, by the increasingly computer coded, shallow, and rationed availability of curative actions imposed by the closing cages of health law and mis-managed care, and by the cancellation of my longest lasting radio program which I realize now was a weekly act of creativity and high joy, as necessary to my needs as my private oil paintings. I did not fit the youthful demographic recommended for stations on the go. Over the years my audience as well as my patients and I had created a very special relationship, weaving hope, faith, and wellness, into a loving willingness to find mutual solutions to our problems. We were no longer free to do so. As much as anything else this book is an effort to reopen that dialogue.

I am far from awakening from this nightmare, yet I am nearer than ever before. Dear friend, don't you see why I am telling you all this? No one can dodge reality! I am rediscovering my humanity slowly. All of us need to do this! I am thinking in terms of "*us*" once more. I am beginning to wonder how many negative experiences have misled all of our minds in the past, how many incorrect conclusions we have failed to question, how many opportunities in disguise were lost, how many times we reacted inappropriately, and how an apparently negative experience might be liberating and perhaps a potential blessing. I was unable to transform negativity and now I'm beginning to wonder if that's not our very first task.

I share the pain of the loss of my son with you because you, my reader, are close to me, and your pain is equal to mine. At moments of weakness or pain we all doubt and we all share our humanity. We find it so easy to scorn or ignore our neighbor, yet we must never forget that our neighbor is our brother and our sister, and death has no respect for our income or our holiness. Sooner or later all of us bear our grief together and what happens to you happens to me. Income, education, class, race, have nothing to do with it. We are all human together at these moments!

In a hospital, the rush and hustle and bustle of blood tests and MRI scans and CT scans, the shouting nurses and secretaries, the busy doctors with their entourages, the other patients and their babbling families, the unexplained police, the bells and loudspeakers, the unhealthy food, all blind us to what is happening today, now, right here, to us!

A modern hospital is no place to prepare for health. With all this chaos and noise around you, how can you keep a picture of the goal of it all in mind? It is too easy to lose our peace in the midst of the complexities. And it is in peace that healing lies. Sometimes the bridge between health and despair is just a good night's sleep.

You may want to stop the jangle first if you are scheduled to enter the hospital, perhaps go into a Retreat and communicate with these vitally important issues within yourself, before going into the chemotherapy, the operation, the $50,000.00 a night bed (sic), and the nurse who wakes you up at 10:00 PM to give you a sleeping pill so you won't wake up and bother the night crew.

Five days after the operation I went home, carrying a majestic number of medicines, to be taken care of by my wonderful wife, who was exhausted.

Since then I have gone over the entire experience many times in my mind. I have discovered the corruption of power in myself. I was a physician and one of the founders of "*The International Academy of Preventive Medicine*," for God's sakes! Don't all those medical people at the hospital realize that I have received "*White House honors*"? Don't the surgeons ever listen to the radio?

With difficulty I have come to realize that the awareness that many people had at that hospital of my position as a fellow physician in their community, and my years of broadcasting, *did* have an effect. Being able to afford a private room, and being operated on by a very high priced prestigious surgeon also had an effect.

The egotistical complaints I have made above no longer hide from me the fact that few of us, reading this, can really expect even that much humanity, humility, caring, or human warmth in a similar situation. It appalls me to realize that my experience was as good as it gets!

# 2

## At War With God

I envy those of you who are secure in your belief. I beg your forgiveness for sharing my doubts with you. Yes, when I was a child, there were moments when I felt I was able to talk with God. I remember being in Manhattan's Central Park on one of those new born stormy days, trudging along with snow up to my hips, feeling a glee and a connection I could not define.

I don't think I'm talking about Santa Claus, nor did I approach this connection analytically, but even at those ages I knew that I must somehow rise above the din and noise. I know I was whole in those moments when something walked along near to me. All my worries, cares, plans, pains seemed healed or healing. I never discussed this with anyone, but I cherished the feeling whenever it overcame me. The bush beside the path became holy to me at those moments.

In the last September before my son died, after a lifetime of his denying any connection with religion or God, I took the young man to Kol Nidre service at his own request. This is one of the most holy sacred services for Jews.

The cantor that evening had first conducted these services at the age of 21, in Auschwitz. He had been warned by the Germans (he had once thought he was a German too) that if he conducted services in the barracks the night of Yom Kippur, he would die slowly of torture the next morning.

He sang his heart out, convinced he was about to die. As he said to all of us, he honored himself, and all around him, on that night long ago. He lived. The Americans were too close. The war was almost over. He had conducted these services every year since, with special prayers for those who did not survive.

He reminded all of us that those who survive are people with courage. People who are disgusted by evil, live an ethical life, and focus on the best in their lives and not the worst, are the ones who live. He reminded us all how frail life is. We must transcend in this moment because there may be no other moments. I wish all of us, Jewish or not, could learn this man's lesson. There were 30 survivors of the Holocaust in the congregation that night.

I expected my son to stay an hour and leave but he stayed for the entire service. The cantor's ethics and beliefs suited his belief system. He admitted in the car going home that perhaps religion does play a role in a better life.

In January I learned I would have to have heart surgery at some point in the future. The support my family gave me at that moment helped me survive the emergency operation several months later, including my middle son's strong hug and his faith in my courage, my power to heal, my strong positives, and in his words, "*the love I offer so many.*"

On March 1st. the van my son was riding in tumbled and rolled, following the bursting of a defective rear tire, and my son died. The van tire blew out because a man did not check it properly, because the van was overloaded with kids coming home from a debate, because my son was asleep without his seat belt on, because the van door lock opened as the van tumbled, because the driver was inexperienced in emergencies, and somewhere I found myself in that equation, as part of the human race. It was not God's fault!

How can others go on in a world of pain and sacrifice? Yet after surgery I was still breathing, with my heart still beating, with my remaining family beside me, with good still in some kind of balance with evil. There came a moment when I remembered that bad things happen to good people. I remembered my dead son at the Kol Nidre service the previous September, and the 30 survivors around us.

There are times when life asks nothing of us except silence, patience, and tears. Plutarch tells us that when Anaxagoras was told of the death of his son he said only, "*I knew he was mortal.*" Maybe I am beginning to understand.

My mother used to quote a German proverb: "*Who has never tasted what is bitter does not ever know what is sweet.*" The game of life is worth the play, but I suggest that the prize may lie in the struggle. There are no winners.

*I have a strange insight. Consciousness comes from suffering. It is those who have suffered who advance the world. Tragedy, difficulty, and adversity are what defines humanity. In crisis you discover yourself. Tears can turn into triumph.*

I am faced by a paradox: We have to fight our "*cancer*" or we will die! If it weren't for hope, our hearts would break. Millennia of witch doctors have taught us that we can choose to die, to stop, to lie down and cease. Whether we live or die is eventually a choice made by our entire being, including the finest, highest, and most conscious part of ourselves. We can't run from weakness. We are all weak. Dear friends, we are alike in the end. We are all capable of doing what we think we can't do, being more than we think we can be, healing what we think can't be healed. We are marvelous, you and I.

I was a grown man and I had been expecting Santa Claus after all. So one sunny day, I once again allowed myself to love, to feel a sense of peace in a garden of roses, at the cemetery, at a motion picture. I laughed again.

Is it any more absurd to believe deity exists in the wholeness of things, than it is to believe that a quark disappears the moment you see it, or that no atom is going to do what all your equations swear it will? I suppose most religious dicta are untrue, yet I see the rose, yet I believe. *Credo quia absurdum est* (I believe it because it is absurd), said the old bigot Tertullian.

I decided to function "*as if*"! Who am I to direct the actions of whatever God there may be, to second guess this vast mystery, to fantasize a large fat man with a white beard and a red suit trimmed in ermine! I hope to be able to function "*as if*" God demanded a certain ethic, a certain morality, a certain human connection. That would be enough. Just for a moment that old companion in the snow was standing near me, knowing my trial.

There may not be miracles, but sometimes there is that fragrance, a sudden shift in attitude that makes all the difference, and it doesn't matter whether we believe in miracles, or even believe in God. We must act as though they both exist, and perhaps we can create them.

To rephrase a wise old saying which is the epigraph to this book, "*We heal each other not because we are sick, but because we are holy.*"

Beloved companion. Draw your servant close to you. My soul is weary and ailing, yearning for your existence and love, asking that You heal me. Reveal Yourself to me, and spread Your canopy over me. Amen

# 3

## My Life

If this book were like my other health books, full of lists and 30-second secrets to health, if all I talked about was vitamins and medicines, then all you would need here would be my MD and my affiliations. For a book like this I owe you a great deal more of myself than that. Besides, I think you will find the child hidden within the physician I am, to be a child much like the child within you. You may even be amused.

I grew up always perplexed. While everything made sense to everyone else, nothing really ever made sense to me. My friends took their purloined Playboy magazine to bed to "*read*," not that I never did, while I began with volume one of the Encyclopedia Britannica, reading the entire set through, including the year books.

I delved into theological and secular issues at the age of 10, making Maimonides one of my idols. Maimonides reminds us to choose life, choose community, and choose love, which as a youngster I learned was a very important life issue. These choices sat well with me. I was a devout believer in the writings of diverse thinkers such as Gandhi; and Heschel, Rashi, and Nachman who are Hebraic; some of the Islamic writers, St. Francis of Assisi who is Catholic, and Lao Tsu, until all their ideas seemed to run so much together I began to have difficulty telling them apart. I found a scientific principle behind the door of almost every religious one, at least I thought so, and vice versa.

I studied at a specialized admittance, university level high school, known as Stuyvesant. You took an exam to get in to prove you were above a certain level of excessive brilliance, where only 14 year old gods like me could go. Calculus and French nearly ruined me.

My dad owned a restaurant. His essence was a cordial connection between the moments of pleasantry. The menu brought joy to most of his clients. He was satisfied.

My parents had full trust in my judgment so I was allowed to use New York subways to travel wherever my interests directed, and I was on the subway alone by the age of nine or so. I visited every single museum, every monument, every bridge, and the great ship Normandy just before it was burned and sunk at the dock by saboteurs.

One summer I went to an Adirondack summer camp. While there, never having seen a hornet's nest, I climbed a tree, in my bathing suit, to bring it down and take it home. It was still occupied. I spent almost three weeks in the hospital. Today I am phobic of bees and insects, and have no desire to lose my fear. Our "*insect friends*" indeed! Bah humbug!

I pleaded with my parents to let me study the trumpet. My mother, of course, had hoped I would study the violin or piano. Dad was hot for the saxophone! The trumpet won out, much to the chagrin of my neighbors. I practiced the trumpet for eight years, with the same dedication I gave to everything else, and ultimately became second trumpet with the Sy Karr CBS Children's Orchestra.

Because Louis Armstrong sometimes dined at my father's restaurant, I got to play "When The Saints Come Marching In," along with him at the Hotel Astor, where he and his band were appearing. He said, "*Boy, you'll be a great jazz player one day, but you need a fancy handkerchief.*" That was the high point of my music career.

I prepared seven months running for my solo appearance with the Carnegie Hall Concert Orchestra. At which time I astonished my parents and myself with a ravaging (or do I mean ravishing?) rendition of the Carnival of Venice, Ave Maria, Angel's Walk, and as an encore, that of course the audience demanded, several Gershwin rhapsodies. I can still hear the applause.

Already being somewhat of a ham I played the role of the "*Mad Hatter*" in "*Alice In Wonderland*" in junior high school, a relatively formal and professionally produced play, that ran three weeks. An agent in the audience got me children's roles on radio soap operas, which I did regularly until my voice changed, and my dad said,

"*Enough!*" Women of a certain age will still remember those kids on the radio soap operas of the time. A lot of them were me.

From the moment I understood the work of my pediatrician, I decided that I'd be a doctor. To me, being a doctor was an impassioned theological act that made a more truthful statement than any religious incantation.

I used the New York Main Library all the while, to read as many books about medicine as made sense to me. I have long known that much of the advantage that certain children have in college is due to this kind of head start.

I recall reading about a brilliant mathematician, newly out of the hinterlands, who wondered how all the other students knew to have notebooks in class, and to take notes. There is so much that is culture and class bound in education. Educated families have no idea of the difficulties faced by the first person in a family to ever go to college.

Then my cousin Lillian died. One day when I was 17, I was picked up at school by my father who told me that my cousin, who was my age and like a sister to me, may have been killed in a motorcycle accident. We had to go to the police department to identify her, and then rejoin the rest of her family who were in shock. I cannot forget my father's tears, or the pain of seeing the body in the morgue. I felt no God, no angel, no voices, no sense of healing, merely pain!

Authenticity and facing sorrow are apparently part of the art of living. Real issues, real experiences, real fears, and now for certain I needed real people.

I graduated from high school with honors here and there. Only three months later I began my freshman year at the University of California at Los Angeles (UCLA) 3000 miles away. I was the angriest freshman in its history. I cast God into hell, if he existed, for His failure to prevent the monstrous injustice, and His failure to spare us the indescribable pain.

I intended to make or break it in the world on my own terms. Such terms included all expenses. Dad only paid the incidentals, such minor things as housing, tuition, and books, which cost a bloody fortune. Yes, I was born with a silver spoon in my mouth. Practically everyone in medical school in America is, then and now.

It wasn't long after beginning at UCLA that I took a job as a salesman part time in a cheap outlet shoe store in Santa Monica, one of Los Angeles' western anchors on the Pacific Ocean. I worked every Friday night and all day Saturday selling Sikonian and Ambrakidian shoes, Nossises, Khian, parrots and hemp soles, saffron mules and around the house slippers, Ionian button tops and night walkers, high ankles, crab claws, Argeian sandals, cockscombs, cadets, and flat heels.

One day I met the president of one of the country's largest steel mills, back when we still had a few left. He came in often. At one point I refused to sell him a remarkably fine Llama calf leather, wing tip shoe, because in my judgment it did not fit and would result in pain and discomfort. He went away disgusted, and came back a week later my fan. He and his wife and I became friends and his letter of recommendation to medical school reached them all.

After my premed requirements were met, I was accepted to all of the medical schools to which I applied. I chose to go on to the University of Southern California (USC) School of Medicine.

I had never faced the issue of religious or other prejudices until, as a freshman, I pledged a medical school fraternity, whose name I will not mention since they are not unique. The night before initiation I received a phone call from a renowned public figure, author, MD, and O.G. of the fraternity. He suggested to me on the phone that it would inure to everyone's benefit, mine included, if I just did not show up at the initiation dinner the next day. He said approximately, "*Your peers are very fond of you, that's clear or you wouldn't have gotten this far. It's just that the elders of the fraternity, well, uh, this is a purely Christian fraternity, and your values are likely to be at odds with ours. Did you know there's a Jewish fraternity on campus? You ought to be joining that.*"

The trauma was significant. My response was, "*If the elders are truly Christian then the only thing you could do would be to open your arms to me. To refuse my membership is to demean the concept of Christianity. But I will not show up tomorrow night, and you can have a good night's sleep.*"

As a boy I came from a neighborhood and school in New York where we all celebrated all holidays and appreciated each other's religions. My class at public grade school was composed of about 35 children, 20 of whom were Jewish, maybe 10 or 12 were Catholic, and the remainder a mix. Other classes had other kinds of mixes. My high school was around 30 percent black. I had never believed enough in the touch and feel of prejudice, even knowing as much as I knew about the world, Bergen-Belsen, the Ku Klux Klan, the Spanish Inquisition, and all that.

A year later I did join Phi Delta Epsilon, the Jewish fraternity, but I never attended their activities, blaming them for what was not their fault really, except that, by banding together as a "*Jewish*" fraternity, they covered over an issue which I thought needed to be brought out and overcome. My parents influenced me in every way they could to hold a human person as a higher value than any other value in life, including the gem stone on the ring of King Solomon.

**Healers need to be creed and color blind.** The singular lie, the "*gentlemen's agreement*", was born for me in my Freshman year at the USC Medical School in the City of Our Lady of Porciuncula, the Queen of the Angels.

Medical school did not come easily to me. With much distress I learned how much easier it was to name an illness than to find a cure, and practice medicine rather than healing. In fact the word "*cure*" became as much a mockery in medical school, or thereafter, as the word "*justice*" has become for lawyers.

My father lay dying of bladder and prostate cancer, aged 53, in the UCLA Hospital at the moment I graduated. We had a private second graduation celebration in his hospital room for him.

There was a great deal of frustration for me in knowing how little cure was available in the 11,000 pharmaceuticals I memorized. My father, attended by professors of mine, received morphine as total treatment for his cancer after I spent four years under their intense tutelage. They asked pompous medical questions on their exams but left my father's cancer "*in the hands of God.*"

Francis Quarles in the 17th. century said,
"*Physicians of all men are most happy; what good*
*success soever they have, the world proclaimeth,*
*and what faults they commit, the earth coverest.*"

I very quickly became a clinical instructor at the USC School of Medicine. In the next year I became Chief of Staff of Westside Hospital in L.A. and Medical Director the year following. That lasted for several years. I also became Medical Director of the American Medical International (AMI) hospital chain.

I met my loving and beautiful wife a few years before we chose to marry, raising three sons, one of which we lost. Our oldest son is presently in attendance at the University of New Mexico, and the youngest is a senior in high school, contemplating university.

I remained in a growing private practice on Wilshire Blvd. My curiosities continued. One of my patients was the dean of a law school. We spent a lot of time arguing about constitutional law. One day he threw the challenge to me, "If you really want to know what you're talking about, why don't you go to law school?"

I attended the University of West Los Angeles School of Law at night for three years. I passed the bar in 1977.

I have always tried to practice my art with mission, with lovingkindness (compassion), and with empathy. I charged a fee for service, but I never really charged more than someone could pay, and often wrote off any charges. I ended many a year, busy as hell, but paying my expenses from last year's savings account.

My name, Gershon, is the name given by Moses to his first son. In Hebrew it means "*Stranger in a New Land*". I have always felt my name to be fitting.

I counseled against surgery whenever I found a viable option, and tried for a very long time with each patient to use the art in place of the prescription, trying to avoid the medicines whenever I had a patient careful enough, and willing, to work along with me. I talked diet, exercise, and vitamins, while the cigarette companies were still telling us that their smoke was good for us

I have a tendency to sermonize. I insist that right is right, and wrong is wrong, although I allow others their right to live in the shaded areas and the shadows! It's big of me, I know.

Pesently I sit outside the working world of medicine but I know I am required to continue on as a teacher, which is what Hippocrates (see Chapter fifteen) taught us a physician ought to be doing anyway.

# 4

## Picking Your Doctor

I was once asked in my dad's restaurant, as a little kid, by a professor of medicine, what I was going to be when I grew up. I said, "*A doctor.*" He said, "*Really?*" I replied, "*Yeah, an ear, nose, and throat specialist*". "*Nose?*" he asked. "*Yeah,*" I said. His comment was, "*Really? Which nostril?*" I didn't know he was kidding at the time. As the years go by I am less and less sure that he was.

Before I get down and dirty, and talk about picking the best possible doctor for us, perhaps I should begin with a controversial word about "*bedside manner.*" How can I possibly be the kind of doctor who can resonate to the deepest levels of others if *I* have become merely the unchanging servant and footstool of their surfaces? I'm a little suspicious of a doctor who seems to be blithely untouched by life. You should beware of a seductive bedside manner. It masks much that is unknown, and much well known (or hidden) incompetence. Lucky is the patient who finds good manners in concert with good medical knowledge. Rejoice.

To further set the stage, I also have something to say about sin, a word you haven't heard very much lately. I remember a real doctor more than 10 years ago, a Marcus Welby type, who lost many thousands of dollars in a suit brought by a clever lawyer for "breach of warranty" since there was no basis to sue for malpractice. It seems the doctor ran into a distraught former patient in the hospital on the way to an appendectomy, kissed her on the forehead, doing no more than promising her she would be just fine - and she wasn't just fine. She had an allergic reaction to anesthesia. She had a semi-stroke, which got better, but she had neurological damage. She had nausea and vomiting.

All the anger at lawyers we see around us today is summed up in that story about a "*clever lawyer*". Even though no laws were broken, that lawyer had sinned. And the patient went along with it! There was evil there, and cruelty. In this regard we often quote Shakespeare, "*First we kill all the lawyers*", and we're only half joking. Something inhuman has crept into our beds and it is best we learn how to remove it as soon as possible. The law is high and ancient, and can be high again.

Many physicians were advised, as a result of that case, never to play the Doctor Marcus Welby role in real life. How many doctors can ignore this kind of thing? We have every reason in the world to be going into surgery scared to death and needing reassurance more than anything else, as I recently discovered. It is the lawyers who forbid that reassurance. When I had my heart valve replaced, I met total human disconnection, and what seemed like glacial coldness. **There is something in the structure of the law that has turned against us and our entire world. It has become a cruel uncaring machine, and is dragging medicine down with it.**

*"An it please ye court: Having 16 years of training, 15 years of medical school teaching, six years of health care for indigents, and 30 years of medical practice, some concurrent, I not being 85 years old, and having been forced to change my moccasins these past few years, specializing now in being a patient, wherefore I respectfully bring to your honor's attention my views of ye component elements entering into a rational choice of personal physician, both from ye doctor's and from ye patient's viewpoint."*

A doctor who is a generalist, who might also happen to be a specialist, is far more capable of seeing our whole picture where our problems usually lie, and less likely to be looking at just our left nostril.

It's likely that the doctor we want is the doctor most other doctors will not want. What I mean by that is we want a doctor who will try to combine basic science, with the perceptions of psychoimmunology, and a healing journey beyond Pythagoras, someone who will see us whole.

We want a doctor who is enchanted by, and satisfied with, standing away from and out of the crowd, not a doctor who is an extension of his charts and rules and facts. Facts eliminate the need to think and understand. They establish only the need to remember.

Beware of Dr. Netmare whose enchantment lies with technology. She will be paralyzed in an electrical failure. She is relieved that it is the process that makes the decisions, leaving her innocent.

Seek a doctor who believes in miracles as well as pills. Seek a doctor who practices standard medicine but understands and respects the values of alternative and complementary medicines, and utilizes them when appropriate. Your doctor should perceive your life style, exercise patterns, diet, attitudes, and psychology.

If you ask an average physician, who has diagnosed a terminal illness, to compile a list of options and methods as an alternate healing strategy, nine times out of 10 she would be totally paralyzed. The textbooks just don't give her any lists and she hasn't done her own thinking.

The physician must use resilience as a healing force, use of thought and process, of lifestyle change, and of prescriptives. The doctor needs to understand that there are cultural differences in medicine.

Love any doctor who has garlic on his breath, despite what Frank Muir said, "*I did not realize what it had done to my breath - one doesn't with garlic - until this afternoon when I stood waiting for somebody to open a door for me and suddenly noticed that the varnish of the door was bubbling.*"

We must know that our doctor has listened to the questions he asked as well as to our answers, and that he has made the effort to explain the process of his thinking to us.

We need a doctor who doesn't always do everything we want, but who can be relied upon with respect to moral values. A doctor must consciously state the truth as she sees it. A doctor who isn't compassionate isn't a doctor.

A teacher of mine said, "*You can't take every patient home to bed with you,*" and yet that's an ancient healing metaphor for the doctor who symbolically must get into an intimate relationship with the patient, and the patient who must issue the invitation. On the other hand I don't think a doctor who carries all her patients on her back is a healthy doctor. The doctor can serve her patient without fusing to the patient. It may be unfair to younger doctors, but we also want an experienced doctor.

Working with our doctor entails more than auditioning potential physicians. We have an important part to play. We might do our part by presenting a medical portrait of ourselves. As I see it there are five main aspects to this portrait:

- 1.) Our past medical history. Our physician will need this in order to be aware of past medical problems, including cancer, heart disease, etc.

- 2.) Our family history, in order to zero-in on possible genetic inheritance, including cancer and heart disease, but also diabetes, high blood pressure and psychological problems including stress.

- 3.) We must have a comprehensive physical examination from head to toe so our doctor can detect an array of medical conditions, from heart murmurs to lung troubles to foot problems.

- 4.) We must review our lifestyle, including smoking, diet, high-risk sexual activities, and drinking. Even simple things such as wearing seat belts and having car air bags must be reported to our doctor.

- 5.) Our "*laboratory values*" (various tests) are critical to our doctor's decisions about us, including a review of our cholesterol, blood pressure, emotions, and stress status. Chemical markers reveal much about overall health. Doc can detect anemias, lipid abnormalities, and much else that might need correction.

We need an aggressive, independent, forceful, free thinking, recalcitrant, non-neutralized doctor who is loyal to the patient

What can be said of these criteria? Obviously they will be hard to meet. A physician has to be smart. He or she has do everything to stay up to date, secure in the new knowledge collected daily, intellectual abilities honed to the best edge possible, with the objective of humane, balanced, and reverent care of others, under any circumstances. Doctor's run from this responsibility too often. They too easily refuse people in need who are complex, either medically, psychologically, or financially. Too many physicians are arrogant.

Conversely, beware of the doctor who has answers for every question. Many physicians learn to relieve worries over life-and-death decisions by developing feelings of infallibility, which are reinforced because their judgment is so rarely questioned. This reflects ego, not intellect. This sense of infallibility may spill over into other aspects of physician's lives. Doctors who fly private planes, for example, have much higher accident rates than other pilots.

Our doctor has to be able to admit that quite often he or she just doesn't understand what is going on with us. We need a doctor who can suspend judgment. You should always seek second opinions in complex or lethal medical problems. This is in your best interest. In the past the assumption made by the insurance companies was that the second opinion assured honesty. Today insurers avoid second opinions because they are expensive. The bean counters only understand first opinions.

While I have enjoyed my 30 years of having patients looking to me alone for medical guidance and expert counseling, it has always been welcome when they told me they wanted to see more than one physician. I have always felt it wise to get several different points of view. I don't think much of medicine as a scientific absolute. The physician should make it easy for us to move to another, perhaps more experienced, physician, to obtain our records with ease, to feel unintimidated, loved, and concerned and cared for, no matter what we decide.

A good test of a physician is the prescriptions he or she is presently writing. They contain powerful molecules. You can ask doc what will happen when you mix three or more of these together, probably not one in ten will go to a computer and check. The others will guess without even bothering to pick up a Physician's Desk Reference (PDR), and they are likely to make the same mal-assumption you will, that if it's prescriptive, it's probably okay. If you are taking several different pills you should be concerned, and so should your doctor.

Doctors can find nothing wrong with more than half the people who consult them. To determine whether the patient is sick, therefore, according to Ian Robertson, both parties commonly enter a subtle negotiation in which each may make compromises in order to reach a mutually acceptable decision. Some patients appreciate a doctor's candor, but others are likely to see it as an admission of incompetence. In such cases, the physician implicitly negotiates a diagnosis with the patient. If the patient refuses all diagnoses, the negotiation has broken down.

Even when a diagnosis is accepted, it must usually be reinforced by a prescription, or patients are likely to feel that they have not received value for their time and money. Just to keep the patients happy, many doctors implicitly accept the patient's suggestion ("*Strep throat*") and irresponsibly prescribe antibiotics, knowing that the condition will probably improve soon in any case. More than half the doctors in the United States admit to having prescribed antibiotics for the viral disease against which these drugs are utterly ineffective, the common cold.

In other cases, patients view doctors resorting to medication as a failure. Even doctors sometimes do, feeling that if they had done a better job, perhaps the patient would have felt better without medication. Everybody has opinions about medicine.

What about your responsibility? The primary care physician we finally choose must know that his patient is genuine. What if she isn't? While the doctor assumes a genuine patient sits before him, he may in fact be facing a white collar thief, or a malingerer. A malingerer can badly hurt medicine, destroy your doctor's faith in humanity, and destroy your doctor.

We want our doctor to understand the difference between irrational concepts on the patient's part, and original and/or unusual ideas and requests. She should have no fear of cautioning us, if we should choose the easy way, instead of the wise way. Our doctor must see the difference between fantasized ills and real ones, still being aware that fantasized ills also need treatment, of a different sort.

Evaluate to what degree the doctor understands that the problem of a patient is the problem of a family. A family can be supportive and curative, or destructive. Even a loving family, left outside in the hallway of the hospital and treated as if they were in the way, is destructive.

Too much of modern medicine is mechanical and unfeeling and becoming more so. Too many patients, as well as doctors, like it that way. You and your family should be partners with your doctor in any discussions of diagnosis, options, and prognosis. You know a great deal about how it feels and what might have caused it, and your doctor is more able to apply his or her expertise, when the information flows both ways. A great deal of medicine is still an art. We are not yet ready for computers to take over.

Every drug has a complex effect on your entire body. Your local public library should have a copy of the Physician's Desk Reference, or you can order it through your independent book store. Every doctor has to have a copy, for legal as well as medical reasons. It lists what is officially known about every permitted prescription drug. The information for some common medications can fill eight pages of very small type. Everything good has a darker side, even aspirin. Do you really want to know the other side?

Will you be intimidated? Somewhere among the extremely rare side effects of almost any drug is listed "*death*". Your doctor may not want you to have all that information if it's going to keep you from taking a quite benign and helpful drug. It's nice to think of being a partner with your doctor in your health care, but you have to realize that it is sometimes a little complicated and you have to bring your mind and spirit along.

Remember that your body is a dynamic system, it is unlike anyone else's, and it can react in new ways at any time. When you take a medication be aware of possible side effects. If you have a tendency to have every disease you read about, learn to discount this. And remember that even a drug you've been taking for years may suddenly turn on you for no discernible reason.

Doc has to decide what level of truth the patient really wants. Being diagnosed with cancer could be a profound personal disaster for you, and you just might not want to know. Doctors spare patients agony in some countries by discussing their findings with the family instead.

It depends upon the patient as to what degree the doctor dares to function. The doctor has to be sensitive to this. He or she is not just thinking of us. In America doctors are ruled more by legal fear than they are ruled by ethics, or lovingkindness.

Many people with terminal illness treasure the time they have left as a chance to put their affairs in order. How many of the rest of us have time to truly say "*Goodbye*" with love and awareness, before we go?

Keeping information from patients "*for their own good*" is in fact a common practice in the United States. Even if you request the information, a doctor may decide that you are unable to cope with truth based upon his assessment of your age, sex, personal history, emotional status, education, etc.

A study in Japan indicated that only 16 percent of Japanese physicians ever tell a patient that they have a terminally advanced cancer. Whereas in Italy less than 50 percent would tell breast cancer patients they had such a situation, and in Spain only 25 percent of cancer patients were ever aware of the true finality of their diagnosis. These cultural myopias may influence statistics.

I feel that the initial manner in which a person reacts to a diagnosis can make it possible for that person to take charge of their life - or totally fall apart, yielding to all the patterns of control by others, accepting, prophesying, and then delivering death.

The patient must take charge, overpower the diagnosis, go to war with it. A physician has to come up with many different options, and present them in a very positive way. A presentation from a doctor in terms of how long you are going to survive, is very manipulative, and mostly is in the physician's interest and not the patient's. They don't want to get caught misleading you, misrepresenting, implying a warranty or guarantee which can get them sued for breach of contract or malpractice.

Despite all of that, you might be surprised to know how far the partnership between you and your doctor can go. You shouldn't have to have a law in lieu of caring, but here are some little known laws that try to give you, by fiat, rights you may have taken for granted:

- 1.) You take your scared and crying daughter to the emergency room of a hospital after a skating accident, and the doctors tell you to step outside while they examine her.

  A: You don't have to go unless they suspect child abuse or if you interfere. If they kick you out anyway, go talk to the hospital's "*Patient Advocacy Office*". Better yet refuse to leave, unless you are obstructing their work.

- 2.) When it comes time for your partner's (friend's, relative's) operation, you want to be there for the tests and consultations. You also want to visit him or her at any time, day or night.

  A: Sure, as long as you are genuinely not in the way. You won't be allowed in the operating room. You belong almost everywhere else.

- 3.) You are changing doctors. Do you get to look at copies of your medical records when they are transferred?

  A: Maybe YES, maybe NO, depending on your State of residence. Check with the "*People's Medical Society*" at (215) 770-1670.

- 4.) You have a car accident while on vacation and you forgot to bring your insurance card with you. Can the hospital emergency room refuse to treat you?

  A: Hospital-YES, Emergency Room-NO, no matter what.

- 5.) When you enter the hospital, they ask you to sign a consent form that absolves them from all liability for everything and lets them do whatever they want forever. Do you have to sign?

  A: No, but they don't have to admit you either. Sign it for minor procedures like taking blood pressure. If they want to go inside your body, through your natural holes, or by making new holes in you, get a new form for each thing they do and make sure you are told the benefits and risks. You get to pick the doctor. The forms are not written in iron. There is room for negotiation. If you do not understand the negotiation, declare that you do not.

- 6.) You want a second opinion. Can your doctor dismiss you for doubting her?

  A: Yes, for any reason. Emergency rooms, and follow-up after an operation, are the only exceptions. So you'd better make sure you have the right doctor from the very beginning. You have a right to know who you're dealing with, so don't pick a doctor who is "*too busy*" to talk. A doctor dismissing you capriciously may be liable for abandonment.

- 7.) They won't let you out of the hospital until you pay!

A: The law calls that "*false imprisonment*" and hospitals can't do it. You can leave at any time for any reason, even against medical advice.

- 8.) When you get the bill, it approximately equals your life savings. Can you refuse to pay or insist on an explanation that makes sense?

  A: Yes (sort of) to both. You have a prior right to an itemized detailed bill showing the $345.00 charge for that aspirin tablet and the $700.00 bill for those three phone calls. At this point you are entering the world of dueling lawyers, and you are on your own. Seek proof of every charge and seek comparable charges to others including those insured differently.

- 9.) The biopsy showed that you had the Big C. If you like to know these things, does your doctor have to tell you your diagnosis and prognosis?

  A: Yes, unless you told him or her not to, or if she thinks you might commit suicide or shoot up the reception room when you find out. The law also says she has to use language you can understand.

I don't want to go to a doctor whose plants are dying in his reception room any more than I want to go to a doctor who doesn't have an object of art in his office, or one who purchased "*Doctor Office Pack 21A*" (complete with 36 inches of unreadable books). That tells me that he sees you as "*Patient Type 21A*" also.

When you are with the doctor, do you see images of healing, or of tire change mechanics? Does your doctor have a talent like an opera singer - or a car muffler repair mechanic? Is he in tune - with you and your music? Is there a common tempo? Is your doctor willing to be aware of the dissonance between your discomfort and your lifestyle? A doctor might argue that, since we take our car in for a checkup, why don't we take our body in for a checkup? My answer is, we don't want to be an automobile! We want our human essence there on the examining table, along with the blood samples.

Doctors may have been bullied into saying that "*I am here to serve you*," but we don't want our doctor to have a "public utility" mentality. We don't want a doctor who will hide behind his white coat, and use our lascivious paper gown as proof of his invincible superiority. We need a doctor who will follow his oath, and not an accountant's flow chart. Even caught up in a crisis, we want a doctor who sees us as a positive challenge rather than as a disaster.

We don't want to be in the hands of a doctor who is enslaved by "*The Standard Practice of the Community*" system, the tort law system that imposes "*no creative thinking,*" or the HMO mis-management system that imposes "*no costs.*"

No one else in all the world has been licensed to commit murder except a physician. Even the judge on the bench cannot condemn people to death merely by telling them that they are incurable. Sticks and stones may break your bones, but words can often kill you. Words have a power stronger than all the violence of the world. Beware a pessimistic doctor. He or she destroys hope. He or she may be expressing incompetence, or ignorance. Who is to say that you will not have a cure, or a remission, for your fatal disease tomorrow morning.

Okay. I've been skating along the edge of an abyss here. Now I'm ready to jump. Hang on.

Medicine does not deal with "*foolproof*" data. In the last few days I have run across three different counts of the number of deaths each year due to infections contracted within America's hospitals. I usually use the smallest figure, 80,000, but it might turn out that the largest is the accurate one: 180,000. At many points throughout this book I have had to choose between conflicting information about the same event. This may be why the word "*suggest*" is so often used in scientific papers in medicine.

Substituting the smaller 80,000 figure in a computation from the Benton Country News Tribune on 17 November 1999, reported on the NET, we get the following startling statistics:

- *Number of physicians in the U.S.*
  *700,000*
- *Accidental deaths caused by physicians per year*
  *80,000*
- *Accidental deaths per physician*
  *0.114*
- *Number of gun owners in the U.S.*
  *80,000,000*
- *Number of accidental gun deaths per year (all age groups)*
  *1,500*
- *Accidental gun deaths per gun owner*
  *0.0000188*

**Therefore -- doctors are more than 6,000 times more dangerous than law abiding gun owners!**

Don't forget that if these 80,000 deaths occurred in any field other than conventional medicine, even this lowest figure would be considered a national disgrace. It amounts to a new Vietnam war every six months.

Stories in our daily paper raise the issue of medicine, death, tort or civil law, and criminal law, and the reality that at least in part, if not in whole, over 80,000 people a year die from mistakes in medical care. Between 40 and 50 percent of the hysterectomies done in America in the last decade were probably not needed! The surgeon was protecting himself against malpractice suits. Malpractice does exist, without a doubt.

Impotence is one of the common complaints received by doctors. Nearly 75 percent of impotence is produced by prescription medicine.

Over 80 percent of ultrasounds done on pregnant women are unnecessary and are possibly dangerous. Their subtle high frequency vibrations may damage the delicate and swiftly growing cells of the baby in some way. Did you know that 50 percent of mammogram results are not valuable? Over 300,000 balloon angioplasties were done in 1990, but there wasn't a single study that showed this dangerous procedure was more effective than prescriptive medicine.

I believe that there are many hundreds of thousands of unnecessary operations performed in the United States every year. There are thousands who are dying from unnecessary procedures and other thousands who have been harmed for the remainder of their lives by procedures they could have done without. The least we should expect is a little humility.

Ian Robertson again, writing in Sociology, has some frightening words for all of us. "*There is no sign whatever that the overall extent of disease is decreasing, even in the emerging societies. No doctor worthy of his or her degrees dares admit that modern medical techniques such as vaccination and antibiotics have had no significant impact on the overall death rate in industrialized societies during the past century! The drastic reduction in deaths is primarily the result of higher standards of nutrition (entraining increased resistance to disease) and innovations in public health, such as milk pasteurization, water purification, food inspection, and insect control.*" Which is not to say that "*modern medical techniques*" don't work. They do.

No wonder medicine is in a state of crisis. The more you learn the more frightening it gets. And look at the many able doctors among us. Can you imagine what's going through their minds? How do you free a physician from his fear of being labeled criminal while you also demand that he or she be creative and consider alternatives, herbal medicine, acupuncture, 4000 year old Chinese or Ayurvedic medicine, yoga, meditation, and the Qi? The "*standard of the community*" is the Merck Manual, Harrison's Textbook of Medicine, and what they said 20 years ago in medical school.

I think its a joke when they tell you that malpractice litigation exists in order to teach doctors how to be more careful, or to create an incentive to improve their quality of medical care. What it does is serve to make the physician more frightened to be daring, creative, thinking, or move even the slightest bit out of the codified, accepted, standard of medical care.

What sorts of un-persons ruling us, so hate the creative, the caring, the spiritual, that all the forces of law and government are mobilized to their destruction? Whose financial motives underlie the destruction of the creative in American medicine and elsewhere? And don't tell me that they don't know exactly what they are doing.

*Perhaps these figures will help you understand how terribly important this chapter is. We must always bring our minds along when we pick our doctor. We must do what we can to investigate carefully who is giving us our health care and even more importantly, who is cutting us, and why. A second opinion, even a third opinion, may be called for in important matters. Take this book along and get into an intense discussion the next time you talk to your doctor. Do some research. Keep your options open. You have a right to informed reassurance at each step of the way. The white doctor jacket is a guarantee of nothing! To what degree does any doctor admit that she is not the primary healer in her own office?*

Is your doctor really willing to talk about phytochemicals, natural diets, beta carotene, the concept of prevention? If you believe that meditation, biofeedback, and relaxation responses are critical to cure, does your doctor know about it? Does he pooh pooh it?

We have a society today that sees a nostril, a thumb splinter, a cataract in the eye, a tumor in the body, but makes no connection with the human who has the problem. Medicine had already failed miserably, before mis-managed care, for the lack of humanity in the relationship. It's going to fail even more miserably now.

Let's look at some examples.

I remember one of my first patients almost 30 years ago. She said, "*They tell me I have a few months to live.*" She told me I looked like a kid. She had colon cancer. "*I'd like to know if it is possible to use my own resources to help*," she said.

I told my colon cancer patient, "*Yes I think you have a lot of things to do*." I changed her diet. I got her off fats. I contacted Linus Pauling who suggested she take between 20,000 and 100,000 units of liquid vitamin C a day until she had diarrhea. She bought ampoules of vitamin C in a pure form, purchased in England. I gave her an occasional injection of this vitamin C at her request.

Pauling suggested I start her on vitamin A. No one was talking beta carotene then. I put her on vitamin E. Adelle Davis had already discussed selenium and I had my patient on selenium. Pauling nudged me to stop as much of her meat diet as she could tolerate and direct her toward a pure vegetarian diet. I pushed her and pushed her, even though you must understand that in terms of 30 years ago that was true quackery, from the viewpoint of traditional medicine.

The lady went back to her oncologist three months later, who expected her to be buried by then, and he found her better, not dead. She worked with me, vitamins, minerals, diet, attitude, meditation (I was a yoga fiend at the time), relaxation, all of the aspects that I am teaching today, and to make a very long story short, this woman ultimately did die of cancer - 11 years later.

AIDS patients, cancer patients, "*terminally ill*" patients, have come to me and said, "*I'm going to die!*" I tell them, "*No you're going to live!*" I don't know whether they are going to live or die, but I start them on the road of faith, of belief in themselves.

I start them on a vitamin program, on a cleansing detoxifying regimen, on a non-fat, vegetarian diet, on a variety of minerals and vitamins, on exercise, on raising self esteem.

**The approaches I have outlined here have brought remarkable success to a large number of patients such as her.**

One of my most memorable patients came to me about 10 years ago. He was in his 50's, having chest pain, angina. We'll call this well known man B.J., which are not his initials. He'd been to cardiologists in New York, Houston and Los Angeles and they all said, "*You need a coronary bypass.*"

Now I want you to read what follows with particular attention because B.J. was to some extent treated generically. If you are at risk or presently suffering from B.J.'s symptoms the chances are good that you would respond positively to B.J.'s regimen. Check with your doctor about this of course.

The man weighed 280 pounds when he should have weighed 170. B.J. was a prime sufferer from Hurry Up Disease, a very wealthy go getter who never stopped, smoked heavily, drank up to a dozen cups of coffee a day, and had a martini for lunch and six for dinner.

B.J. told me, "*I heard you on the air and I heard your posturing that there are options to invasive cardiology that may be in the works. You talked about some studies in Japan. You talked about some observations in your office. I want to become involved.*"

I replied, "*You know, what concerns me B.J. is, that if you have been to a bunch of cardiologists then you have to understand,*" and here's the medical/legal disclaimer you see, "*that you are facing the problem, and so am I, of interfering in the standard customary practice of the community. It's possible, but not absolute, that you might be able to reverse your medical situation. I'm willing to give it a try if you and your family are willing to come in here and sign a paper that says, "This is your election.*"

"*According to what you tell me, you've got something like a 75 percent stricture in two important blood vessels which raises the risks significantly for you. If we don't get you treated in some way, you'll have a coronary.*"

I laid out all the risks for him, and said, "*I want you to understand that we are not facing the known. We're going to be facing the unknown possibilities together. The standard practice in the community at the present time is to take you in and absolutely do a coronary bypass.*" B.J. replied, "*I'm not going to do a coronary bypass, so either I die or you help me to get better, but those are the only two options I am selecting.*"

He had to get into a completely different eating style. I allowed him a glass of red wine every night because he wanted alcohol. At the time I did not know the theory that red wine was potentially valuable for helping heart disease. I cut all fats from his diet except the high omega 3 containing fat of fish for dinner four days a week. Breakfast was to become fresh fruit and oatmeal. Lunch was to become a vegetable salad with two teaspoons of olive oil and any fresh juice (O.J. for B.J.?), and the rest plain water. There was no more caffeine. There was no alcohol for lunch.

I said to B.J., "*Options might be a pasta which is boiled plain with vegetables boiled plain, or in a Chinese restaurant, salt free steamed vegetables with occasional steamed shrimp which, while they have cholesterol, also have chemicals in them which help raise HDL. There will be no cheeses. There will be no fatty dairy products. It is truly totally non-fat except for the fish and the olive oil. It is white of eggs, omelet or poached only since nothing can be fried, on dry toast for lunch.*"

In terms of an exercise program I said, "*We're going to begin by walking one block daily, if that's comfortable. If not, half a block. When we are comfortable with that, every three weeks we'll add another half block. We're not in a hurry. We're just going to take a walk that's relatively regular. Every three weeks as long as there are no symptoms, we're going to add an additional half a block.*"

"*You're going to take 10 minute breaks four times a day during which time you're going to get into meditation.*" I taught B.J. meditation. "*You're to stop the telephones, four of them ringing every 40 seconds, while you're doing something else. You're going to tell your secretary that telephone time is 10 minutes at the end of each hour at which time you will take calls and return calls.*"

I said, "*You will close shop at 6:00 PM. You will go home. Whatever business you had been attending to will end. If it doesn't end B.J., you will die! You will get involved in intellectual and genuinely pleasant pursuits, family oriented, theater oriented, education oriented, or quiet music oriented. Your music will be lovely classical, no more pop rock.*"

"*When you get into the car you'll plan on listening to music and you'll plan on driving at half the speed. You're going to have to get used to being happy rather than being right. You won't be listening to screaming news and traffic patterns. If somebody cuts you off on the highway, you're no longer going to speed up and give them the finger and almost kill both of you.*"

It was a lot of work working with this guy. I was half convinced that he really should have his coronary bypass because I was worried about his compliance. I have given similar advice to other patients over the years and all the rest of them have, to some extent at least, failed to follow my regimen and advice, whether their life depended on it or not.

B.J. was magic. He actually did comply. He began affirming that he was worthy of a different life. His family reported that he was a new man. He stopped screaming. He started out about as hostile as you could get, Type-A personified. He gave it up. He became loving, even to his employees. He started sending flowers, giving gifts, getting involved with church activities, volunteering. He took up painting in the evening. He never turned the television on any more. He got many more hours of rest because he no longer worked until 10:00 PM, ate and drank until 12 midnight, and slept from 1:00 AM to 6:00 AM.

Within a matter of three months his anginal chest pains disappeared. His blood pressure normalized. His weight came down dramatically. Within a year's time he was down to about 185 to 190 pounds.

He flew back East, without telling me, to see one of the cardiologists he had seen before, who was shocked to find him walking around the way he was, looking the way he did. Unknown to me he got another angiogram. I never got to see it, but I am told that his former 75 percent lesion was now just short of being a 50 percent lesion. The doctor told him, "Whatever you're doing, keep it up."

I saw him in a restaurant about three years ago and I was ashamed of what I was eating compared to the way he ordered. He could have brought partial compliance with our regimen, a massive heart attack, and a malpractice suit into my office. Instead he brought his mind as well as his heart condition. He brought life!

On the other hand I have no intention of trying to be a faith healer. God may not have cure in mind this time. God is also known for helping those who help themselves. My patients helped themselves with vegetables, fruits, omega 3 fish oil, selenium, beta-carotene, exercise, belief in self, meditation, faith in the ability of the body to heal, and if they believed, faith in God. I tried to give all of my patients who had been told they were terminal, specific goals to follow every day, to keep them busy getting better, thinking better, affirming themselves. The secret of survival is maintaining hope.

On the other hand, fear can motivate us. You never stop smoking until they start talking cancer. You never lose the 30 pounds until you discover your blood pressure is elevated. When you fear a possible heart attack, it focuses the mind marvelously.

Now please allow me to speak more generally and a bit more philosophically about your relationship with modern medicine.

In the 16th century Paracelsus said, *"The physician should speak of that which is invisible. Anyone who is not a physician can recognize illness from symptoms, but this is far from making him a physician. He becomes a physician only when he knows that which is unnamed, invisible and immaterial, and yet has its effect."*

I'm not sure how you would move those words into an angiography room, or an MRI scan room, or a room where the doc's only words to you are, "*Come back in two weeks and we'll talk.*" We want a doctor who will bring fantasy, imagination, and his own humanity to our needs. We want to understand that we are not alone.

The hospital is the enemy. We want a doctor who will understand that. The moment we grant spirituality to the human body it becomes an inexhaustible collection of signs. A modern up to date medical textbook and an ancient and wise textbook written by Hippocrates or Paracelsus may be equally important to your health.

The kind of medicine I advocate probably existed once when Hippocrates walked the earth, and it has probably existed through the millennia among the medical men who still quietly carry on, outside the spotlight. I don't want to imply that there are no efforts to improve the situation today. One physician's group, promoting personal awareness among physicians, advocates a curriculum including four new "*core*" topics, including physician's beliefs and attitudes, physician's feelings and emotional responses, challenging clinical situations, and physician self-care. They point out that too many physicians learn difficult lessons in solitary reflection or by chance discussions in hallways or cafeterias, or even through professional censure or malpractice litigation.

Many years ago I knew an Indian medical man in New Mexico who told me that White Men will never really come to terms with cures and healing until they are able to hug a tree, commune with a rock and listen to a blade of grass. He really said that! His wisdom came from the earth (and possibly from a lot of hippies who passed through on their way to Lhasa). Perhaps we should begin to listen to the "*eco freaks*" and the "*tree huggers*".

I recall one doctor I had called into consultation because of unexpected problems. While the doctor was speaking, the patient had quiet Gregorian chant on in the background. The doctor asked her to turn it off. She refused, saying, "*I need that Gregorian chant. It helps me meditate. It helps me feel free and secure.*"

The doctor told her that she could feel "*free and secure*" 20 minutes from now. He needed her total attention at that moment. I don't want a doctor like that. I've made more prescriptions for patients to listen to Gregorian chant than I've made prescriptions for penicillin.

Henry Thoreau wrote in Walden, *"I rejoice that there are owls. Let them do the idiotic and maniacal hooting for men. It is a sound admirably suited to swamps and twilight woods, which no day illustrates, suggesting a vast and undeveloped nature which men have not recognized."* If all a doc is focusing on is our tennis elbow, and he hasn't learned that we need to hear Thoreau's (and Athena's) owl, then he is not the doctor for us.

I believe strongly that a great deal of the success of older healing traditions is probably due to their still undissolved connection between the healer and the healee. The Indian medical man, chanting, dancing, drumming, fasting, laying on feathers and smokes and salves and hands, is an intimate part of your condition at every step. His lack of modern sophisticated and scientific medicine is in large measure made up for by his personal and physical involvement with the patient. After that kind of total sensory overload, you wouldn't dare get worse!

Ayurvedic Medicine, the ancient medicine of India, is influencing traditional Western medicine in many quarters. This is why someone like Depak Chopra is so respected today. I missed seeing this dimension when he was on my program.

Now I see him as combining his religion with medical information. I'd rather have a religious doctor, as long as he doesn't impose his specific religious beliefs on me, for the simple reason that he is more likely to express moral imperatives.

Years ago you were angry at the suggestion that you might have a "*psychosomatic*" illness. Today we are learning that all illnesses are, to some extent and almost by definition, "*psychosomatic*." You need a doctor who understands the connection between a psychological event and a physical ailment.

When truth is absent there is no healing. Failure can often be merely lack of experience, not a failure of technology. As I have often said on the air, destiny can often just be mismanagement. Experience can lead to authenticity and truth.

The true healer's spirit and intuition must be involved as well as his shining apparatus. Is your healer afraid to express his (or her) emotions? How about us? Are our hearts and minds locked? We fear that emotion makes us too vulnerable. It is too easy for those men as well as women, who have trained themselves to be "*dispassionate*" and "*scientific*", to express themselves through an order for a CT scan, a blood test, a 21 gauge needle, and an EKG.

Be gentle in your turn. Your doctor is feeling hard pressed these days. The government and the insurance companies have him or her by the throat, and your anger and frivolous lawsuits might just drive your physician into becoming a stock broker or even, God forbid, a writer. We need all the good doctors we can get.

If a doctor is an empathic, loving, caring person, he or she grieves when a patient dies. A doctor may not have the coping mechanisms that others have. He may feel isolated, aggrieved, guilty, worried about not doing better. Death during the doctor's care is a tremendous stress to the doctor as well. Empathic doctor's are emotionally impacted when something goes wrong and they need to tell grieving friends and family.

Some doctors are going to break under the pressure. Many doctors, unknown to patients, are beginning to have occupational diseases caused by the incredible pressure on them, and the need to worship new gods as well as the gods of healing. In addition to responsibility for the life and health of patients, tensions result from uncertainty about clinical management, the legal and family aspects of health care, and correct medical care. There are long and uncertain working hours, seven days and nights a week on call, and problems involving personal relationships with patients, which on the one hand we say are necessary, and on the other hand can turn bad. These are all imposing almost impossible demands.

Alcohol abuse, chemical dependency, domestic violence, physical and mental illness, are problems that physicians are now encountering in their private lives as well as in their practices. Doctors are at risk.

Examination of the unclothed patient has a potential for a sexual response in some doctors, and there are threats of malpractice litigation every time you walk into a patient's examining room. There is easy access for doctors to addictive drugs or alcohol, or both. Doctors are finding it increasingly difficult to maintain the cultural and economic environment (that expensive house and glossy car) which tradition leads them to think is expected of them. The public is right to be concerned about physician behavior. These are issues that must be aired.

Does your healer have time for this kind of talk or understand it? Most will say, "*No. Get thee to the echocardiogram and leave me to rush off to the next examining room and the next patient. I have a home to pay for!*"

A great American Indian medical man, Chief Silver Bear, taught, "*When you walk in darkness, it is no use carrying a lantern whose light cannot be seen. It might cause you to trip or stumble, or abandon the journey. You must always carry a lantern bright enough for the way you have come and are going so that the way may be marked and hold no fear. You will walk with assurance, leaving yourself no chance to grope in the dark. Be a sun, and become well.*"

*It has been a contagious march, this thing called science, of the greatest arrogance and worth. It has eliminated the ineffective poultices, salves, unguents, decoctions, and poisons, of ancient leech-craft, but we must not look to science for concern and love.*

The people I have had the most success with are those who have liked me, I have liked them, and we don't know why. There has been a willingness to trust each other, a willingness to allow each other our vulnerabilities, a willingness not to expect cosmic certitude from me, and a willingness for us to be partners. It is in that kind of environment that I have been able to work best with people. Those who created a god-in-white were the ones who stayed sick.

In my office I wore my white *"doctor jacket"* at first until I began to realize that patient's blood pressures were much closer to normal if I took my jacket off. I stopped wearing it. I ultimately walked around in a white shirt and tie, so that people could see me as a human being.

Is all this easy to do? Don't be funny! It's almost impossible to find a doctor who suits all of your needs. The best start is probably referrals from friends and patients, rather than other doctors, or those television ads God forbid! We should know by now that the truth is not in television. Doctors tend to refer based on friendship, or comfort working with each other, and not necessarily based on the best thinker or doer on our behalf. Start looking for a doctor when you are well.

Can you find another doctor? Do you really have a choice? Yes, if you are wealthy. The rest of us, relegated to the health insurance debacle, and a shrinking pool of independent doctors, probably do not. You have no idea how sorry I am to say this. I have used the word "*crisis*" often in this book, but never with more urgency. A crisis is what we are facing in America, and in more than health care. The conclusion is obvious, although I can't bear to face it.

Before I conclude this chapter with some remarks about a taboo subject in America, may I remind everyone reading these words that we are all halting, incomplete, and partial, all capable of growth. We are a possibility, a frail reed, subject to revision, barely rational. We join all men, and all human history, in our quest for healing, and finally end up defining humanity in our effort to cure our ulcer, or our heart. "*I am not a number! I am a free man!*" cries John Drake at Portmeirion.

Communication is a two way road. We often blame the doctor for not hearing our problems without realizing that we really haven't presented them. Our denial can last all the way to, and into, the doctor's office even though our purpose in paying that visit is being ignored.

And so, finally, I need to mention a hidden corruption underlying my words throughout this book, which few of us will detect. I painfully realize that I am not talking to everyone. I am talking to a middle class audience in this book. Many unsophisticated people are so used to vocabulary overload from print, that they have learned not to use that source for information.

On the rare occasions when a book is verbally simple enough to be understood by relatively uneducated people, the author too often assumes that they are childlike, or stupid, and is so condescending to them that they can only be mystified or angry. Nonverbal people are not necessarily stupid.

Like it or not, there is an underclass in America and they don't know how to talk like we do. They have been persuaded, by a lifetime of being told to shut up, that everyone above them knows more than they do, even about themselves. Their interactions with authority are based on unquestioning acceptance. They have no idea what a "personal physician," or "my lawyer," or "my broker" might be. They are truly open only to their peers. Any discussion at all, across class lines, leaves them mystified and silent. No wonder they are so silent in the doctor's office. No wonder a doctor must jump to conclusions too often.

Discussion of class is taboo in America because it goes against our collective myth of equality, but it is certainly one more area where our search for healing must go. A doctor who does not take the time to get to know his patients may be unconsciously writing a good and worthy share of the human race out of medicine altogether, as they have already been written out of the political process.

- *Sidney Wolfe. "9,479 Questionable Doctors."*

- *Naifeh and Smith, "The Best Doctors in America."*

- *The Joint Commission on Accreditation of Healthcare Organizations - (708) 916-5800.*
- *HMO accreditation information, National Committee for Quality Assurance - (202) 628-5788.*

# 5

## The Still Small Voice of God

The next subject is religion. In fact it is *theology.* I invite you to hold my hand and dance into this discussion with me. You may not realize at first that you have been down these roads before, on your own. It's not so bad. And ultimately the subject is still your health.

In the past philosophers taught that all of reality could be broken down into four elements. They were right. The four elements of our everyday human reality are still Earth, Air, Fire, and Water (EAFW) or as they were for the Romans; Terra, Aer, Ignis, Aqua (TAIA). Yes I know that scientists have filled the periodic table with well over 100 "*elements*", but they are talking about something else. EAFW are what I mean by "*the deep basis of our reality*". They are a vivid and true poetic metaphor.

Let me explain. Consider EAFW as a simplifying way of remembering - a mnemonic. We may find it a lot easier to think about everything in our world without losing our way if we look at EAFW this way.

What it means to be human is not a matter of science or technology. Insight and human truth have been available to us from the dawn of civilization. The spiritual strivings of the great founders, Jesus, Muhammad, Buddha and all the others, were no less deep than ours today just because they lacked motorcars and airplanes.

These holy ones bring strange tales back to us. Unless we can admit that something unusual has happened to these people it would be ridiculous for an intelligent person to credit their stories. They seem to be trying to explain an extremely unlikely experience, a most surprising product of the human brain. At the core of the world's religions, within the true self, at the core of the soul, is said to be an experience of undifferentiated wholeness. Perhaps Man must speak before God does. "*Let there be miracle! Fiat Deo!*"

Science has just begun to realize how much chaos still flows through God's continuing creation. The butterfly takes wing, and the resulting hurricane kills our mother. For better or worse we are, and always have been, co-creators with God.

The dirty confrontations of our world gain meaning in this context. We must learn that both sides of many current arguments are valid, depending upon where you stand. What authority should government have to legislate morals? Do we have authority over the body or mind of our sister? Are we really entitled to our own opinions? Must we behave as if we were, in order to keep our society from falling apart? This and a hundred other debates surround us and bedevil us today. We need a connecting and spiritual vision, a clear road to travel. We need a way to pray.

And so we come to the great dreams of humanity. May I say once again, it will help if you realize that what follows is poetry and metaphor, and not necessarily literal truth.

The Greeks and Chinese saw EAFW, the Hebrews saw four letters, the Tibetans four implications, but all tied them together and saw ultimately the same reality. The world was formed by the letters pronounced - the "word" - the logos of God. I know that I have changed the traditional order these elements are presented in a couple of cases

In Hebrew the first (sic) letter of the creation of the world is "*Hay*," which means body, as contrasted with the Greek and Chinese word for earth,, the Tibetans called it function, while everyone believed that it reduced to "*doing*," or "*behavior.*"

The repeated second letter ("*Hay*") of creation also means mind. For the Greeks and Chinese it was the equivalent of air, and to the Tibetans it meant creation. "*Hay*" is ultimately "*knowing*".

In the Hebrew description of the creation of the universe there is the third letter "*Yod*," which means spirit, the equivalent of the Greek and Chinese idea of fire, and the Tibetan idea of emanation, but all of them can be defined ultimately as the word "*intuition.*"

The fourth letter, "*Vov*" which means heart, is translated water in Greek and Chinese, although also viewed as heart. The Tibetan Buddhists saw this as formation. "*Feeling*" is what everyone meant by this.

For all, these four supernal words were meaningful because they were an involvement of the human mind with suffering, and the creation of the worlds: the world of doing, the world of knowing, the world of intuition, and the world of feeling. You can see that every part of our life can be described by one or more of these four, EAFW. **This is the great filing system of history**.

Some Buddhists also add the element of space, and the element of emptiness, one of the origins of the concept of zero. *Being or nothingness* is sometimes considered to be the ultimate question. All that exists can be described by zero and one, as any computer programmer can tell you.

Prayer or meditation, whatever word we care to use, is the vehicle we use to travel the road between the elements of life. Prayer has never been labeled as Lutheran, Greek Orthodox, Buddhist, or Egyptian.

Until recently, prayer in a hospital associated with a doctor and a patient, was considered eccentricity. Suddenly we are now encouraging patients to pray. It's not difficult to see how prayer involves EAFW. Prayer doesn't require logic. It doesn't require mathematics. Microscopists will never anatomize prayer, any more than geneticists can ever fully describe why the frog behaves like a frog. That is not to say that we can heal solely at a pure level of prayer. We also need mindfulness, discipline, and scientific fact.

When you add it all together the hard question then is, if prayer is shown to ensure a better chance for us of avoiding or healing cancer, is it that or is it our own body messages, or angels, or cleansing and detoxification of our bloodstream that does the work? Is this mysticism or is it neuroimmunology? Does it matter?

Now please allow me to include traditional American Indians in this discussion because I think the shamans have something to say. Many traditional Indians believe in giving away a negativity, not denying it, but being careful not to send it to someone else, so that communicable diseases, for instance, are sent somewhere where they are transformed into their positive opposite. In this way they encounter the cyclical nature of the world, the great circle of the seasons, the hoop of life.

Transforming sickness in this way, changing greed into generosity, changing envy into self esteem, producing richness out of simplicity, may be the secret to health. Yin and yang, the dances of Shiva, are the same insight. They are seldom heard of in the three great Middle Eastern religions, Islam, Christianity and Judaism which deny duality, and attempt to destroy the shadow half of reality (Satan). In my opinion this is a mistake because it cannot be done.

The Indian concept of the circle of life includes all that was, all that is, and all that will be, with an undifferentiated infinite at the hub, the "*nave of nothingness*". The Indian shaman says that out of a no-thing comes all things. So do the Christian mystics. The circle is sacred to many Indians because it is an entry to understanding themselves, an entrance into life, an entrance into death, and a willingness to accept and meet them both in harmony. Nothing ends. Einstein and Buddha said it and the Indian healers say it. Matter/energy is never destroyed or lost, only transformed.

An Indian example is an apple cut in half crossways. There is a five pointed star within. Within the star, from which the apple has grown, is an empty space. That emptiness symbolizes "*the thing*" that then manifests as all the opposites of reality, another way of saying God.

Western materialism has its basis in a simple physical explanation for all absolutes. An American Indian medical man (and many others around the world), may say that what is seen has its source in that which is unseen and, conversely, that the visible is part of the source of the invisible.

There are many elements in the traditional Indian version of EAFW. Part of what we need to do, they say, is use the power of all four directions, the power of knowledge, clarity, enlightenment, awakening. What follows would be modified of course depending upon to what tribe we are talking. And don't forget that I am describing a powerful metaphor here, not necessarily any kind of objective reality.

To the East is the journey to find new life for ourselves. Out of the East comes the element of fire, oxygen, clarity, and the energy of light. The Sun is born every day in the East. As fire cools it becomes elemental water.

The Southern part of the wheel becomes the lower part of the body placing water there in one sense, while the earth gives us solidification, stabilization. To the South is the power of knowledge, truth, love, trust in our intuitions connected to our spirit, the womb, growth. That's where we get close to matter. If we look to the South, we are able, according to the Indian, to find the things that cause us our pains and discomforts, so that we can let go of them. We free ourselves from the encumbrances and the baggage we carry.

As we move to the North, we move toward knowing. Here we manifest visions of ourselves. Here we take our creative ideas, our thoughts, and we produce actions that are derived from them, which can bring about the desirable changes we want in our life. As we journey to the North, we find ourselves less a victim of circumstance than ever before, less willing to claim that we are ruled by destiny. We are less a puppet of the world around us, and we come to realize our wisdom, the full nature of ourselves. The North contains the power of renewal. Air blows at its strongest from the North.

And on to the West where we examine the ability to change and face the reality that death is part of life. When we have learned that death is not an ending but a transition, then we are more nearly able to give up fear which causes so much of our suffering. We can contemplate new directions, new illuminations. In the West we gain strength, and examine ourselves. It is here we look for change within, transformation, introspection, the setting sun, completion.

"*The Center*" the Indian calls our soul. The quality of the soul is trust and innocence, which is necessary for greater health. Innocence means the yielding up of suspicion and cynicism and materialism, keeping our childlike anticipation. There is a faith that all things will be good. The Indians teach that we hurt our soul with each trauma, rape, divorce, mugging, accident. Every time we let someone else make our decisions for us we give away part of our soul. They say that a lot of our diseases are caused by loss of soul, and therefore a loss of energy and power.

As Westerners we tend to think of Indian healing practices as fostering transcendence, taking us out of themselves. This is incorrect. For us, the Indian vision quest must seem to take place within our Western Cartesian grid, a mandala, in order for us to be able to "find our way back" afterwards. This is exactly not what the Indian is doing. He does not want to find his way back. Wherever the ritual takes him is the right and balanced place for him to remain.

Throughout this book I am asking the healer and the patient to welcome some kind of powerful force into the process. At times I use the word God. It has been inevitable that I do so. There is a need for comforting, and an emotional welcome within humanity, that seems to demand such an idea whether it is "*objectively*" true or not. I hope that the poetry of EAFW has meaning for you. I have been walking these roads for a long time in search of meaning in my own practice of medicine, and in my larger life.

I have no proof, and I hope for truth, but I realize that the world does not, will not, and probably cannot, give the certitude I ask. I study the world's mystic traditions to find wholeness and yet my own life is only confusion. I must find the way for myself, as must we all, if what we find is to have meaning for us.

And so I came to it:

**On a dark night, as I struggled to deal with my physical and professional chaos and make sense of the death of my son, I wondered if I had asked for the correct partner in the healing process. In the blackness I wondered with fear and loathing if a choice of prayer to "*God*" might even take my genuine options from me. Could it be that I am merely imposing a finite set of rigid standards on the mystery of healing?**

**What do the four directions and the world's traditions have to do with me, now, here? I claim that fear and guilt is at the base of most illness and in my night I begin to doubt. Am I increasing the patient's guilt, not removing it, when I dream of a God's infinite healing?**

**We see everywhere in the world, now and always, the conflicts the concept of God has induced. Where has it mitigated the brutality, the vulgar ugliness? And if we say things would be far worse otherwise, what are we then saying about the nature of mankind - and thus of ourselves?**

**Have I asked us, on these pages, to accept a subtle Santa Claus into our souls? A placebo named Santa Claus may heal if we welcome and seem to need it. Are we children?**

A nightmare presented itself to me that night when I pressed for the imposition of God and spirit. Could it be that we have taken the patient, and healing, farther from clarity in our search for meaning? Could we be moving away from, not toward, what we call the truth? Are we all falling into a maelstrom of confusion?

This historical baggage includes standards upon standards, which may produce conflicts upon conflicts, that conceivably could entail illness and not health. As I present the old structures of holiness, are we being overwhelmed with systems of nonsense embedded in the ancient writings and traditions, and the world of print and electronic media?

I fear I may be geometrically increasing the nonsense and chaos of our ill health. In the end am I giving us terror, not peace?

On that lonely night I was more and more convinced that each and every one of us lives in and with fear at all times, generic or focused, or both. I know I will never again be unfearful of a gun in my face. I will never again be unfearful of an exploding right-rear tire. All of my fears are born of my thought and imagination, and my memory. They come from all that I am. They may come from, and be part and parcel of my humanity!

My night continued with the question: Is the choice between life - and nothing - a real choice? What price must we pay? I haven't the slightest idea what human life is all about. No one ever has.

We live in the illusion, or the delusion, that our eternal wars and atrocities are not intrinsic to human nature. We live in hope and no certain truth. What decision can be ours?

In my confusion I asked us all to indulge in faith. I believe it is a factor in healing. Yet I know that traditions from the centuries, and religion after religion, impose faith! They outline, standardize and define us, and our lives. They have determined our behavior, our minds, defined our guilts, listed our conflicts and our limits. We do not own ourselves. They own us!

I cannot stop the flow of thought as I lie awake staring into the darkness. I get up in the quiet of the night, turn on the light over my desk and start writing. Do our traditions of faith, and our religions, rob us of free action, rob us of imaginative and creative movement, that might in fact heal us, and society? How can we ask our patient to think for him or herself when we impose the rigid bars of tradition, rule, and religion?

If the doctor must heal within the "*standard practice of the community*," he or she is also captured by the ancient community of faith in addition to the chromium community of medicine, by the usual, the inevitable, the memorized standards, the always expected.

This book pleads with the healer to be original. How is it possible? The beliefs, standards, and practices of the community deny the world as it is, in spite of us!

How can we work with reality? Would this make us free? And if free, less afraid, and if less afraid less angry, and if less angry less guilty, and so perhaps more effective and thus in transcendence, despite the absent God?

We preach hope, but within ourselves we fear to know that hope is hopeless, because our standards and imposed cultural and religious programming, our theologies and training, have defused hope and made it unreal and impossible.

Truth has no prior program. Truth is not a static way. In my night I ask, what in medicine that is static can heal anything?

We ask desperately for religion to lead the way, yet we know in the darkness that it has caused the most hate, the most anger and fear, the most pain and suffering. Does it lead anyone anywhere? Does it not follow instead? All religions rise in pain, in sorrow, in disbelief and agony - in war! How can we depend on God?

Can it be that I am recommending fictions in this book? Are we programming readers as they read us?

Until we leave the level of the absurd, of hate, brutality, ugliness, guilt, anger and fear, we are dead! I rediscover an awareness, as the sky begins to lighten on my night, that we can indeed not be healthy alone. We need others, in order to be well. We need to change.

**We must allow, and cause, the sun to rise. Without our own change, and change in our society, there is only death, but how do we change amidst yesterday's conflicts imposed upon today's? We are programmed to lie. Is such a dark night a necessary part of our journey? Perhaps we must fight for every foot of our way.**

I returned from my night journey with some hope. We cannot live in the heights or the depths. We must have a place to stop. The horns and buzzers must be stilled. Sometimes we must step off the road for awhile. If we are to remain sane and healthy, in today's world, we must make a quiet place for ourselves where the sun may quietly rise, and we may hear the song of the dawn.

No job, no government, no technology, no religion, is bearable if it leaves us no resting place. We need a place where no one can disturb us. I'm describing a home. I am describing church and temple. When fear and anger overcome us, we can only head for our contentment space for solace.[1]

These sacred places may be our own discovery, sacred only to us. Sometimes a sacred location resides only in our memory. The green and golden days of our childhood may return, to be there when we need them, all through our life. Sometimes still I walk, no longer alone, through the bright snow of Central Park.

Environment has a profound effect on our mentality, mood, emotion, and spirit. If you're not religious, put a rose in a vase, or whatever will induce peace in yourself. Buy a wooden wall shrine (butsudan) from a seller of Asian religious supplies and decorate it with your own symbols. We look for inspiration in a locus, a place, whether it's out on the lake, carefully not catching fish, or looking into the flame of a candle. Dean Ornish used a closet for this purpose earlier in his life, which became a sacred shrine for him.

Studies show that people who regularly attend some form of worship service tend to be in better shape and live longer. Skeptics might say we are confusing correlation with causation. So? Churchgoers may simply have better health habits, have larger social circles, or feel more social pressure to walk the straight and narrow.

I tend to feel that the most important element throughout all of this is humility, something in terribly short supply. Our definitions define us.

In recent studies of Americans 55 and up, meditation was found to be an effective treatment for high blood pressure, lowering it as much as medication did. Dr. Andrew Weil has furnished his clinic in Tucson with fine wood furniture, not chrome. The lighting is low and music is piped in. The atmosphere is relaxed. We're beginning to learn.

"In the meditative state, one feels a kind of expansiveness. Yogis would understand this as a feeling of unity, as the true state of existence, and think of the separation of the self from the rest of the world as an illusion."[2]

In I Kings 19:11 it is said, "*And, behold, the Lord passed by, and a great and strong wind rent the mountains, and brake in pieces the rocks before the Lord; but the Lord was not in the wind; and after the wind an earthquake; but the Lord was not in the earthquake: And after the earthquake a fire; but the Lord was not in the fire: and after the fire a still small voice (kol demamah dakkah, the sound of delicate silence).*"

Healing is the focus where everything in us becomes united in life and everything that is fragmented rejoins, becomes whole. All that we are, our soul, is manifested in reality, for we have come to recognize our mortality. In healing we sanctify each new moment within our lives. This is transcendence, nowhere written in materialism and technology.

We need not ask ultimate questions and expect answers. We may not be connected to objective truth. Even so, spirituality can provide us with a sense of connectedness. It is something that medicine drastically lacks. We miss it. We feel that we must care for each other. We must come together in those moments of meaning. We need a spiritual encounter when we are ill, consciously or not. A doctor has the same need in attempting to heal others.

*We are so insignificant, yet we sense that we are*
*caught up in something infinitely greater than*
*ourselves, a significant power, and we an integral part*

*of it. We despairingly hope that we can become a meaningful part of it as well. True or not, the hope does us credit, and gives us what nobility we can claim for ourselves, in this world of power and privation, meat and murder.*

I remember when I was in grade school, Fulton J. Sheen, not yet a bishop, saw nine of us from school. I was the only Jewish student. Everyone bent their knee except me. He asked me why. I told him I was Jewish and "*We don't do that.*" He said, "You're Jewish, in a house of God, without a yarmulka? You should know better than to enter the house of the Lord without your head covered." He sent an assistant at once to get me a cap.

He asked me to recite the Shmah, the prayer of entry into the synagogue. I told him "I don't know it." He then had me repeat after him, as he recited the old Hebrew prayer. He told me he wanted me to return in two months knowing it by heart.

He asked me if I thought God would mind if an old man blessed a young boy? Scared to death, I told him that I didn't think so. He told me to bow my head but not my body. I did, and he blessed me, and then told me to go over and sit in the chair while he took care of the eight Catholics. It was a remarkable lesson in love and theology and tolerance. All my life I have been able to find moments of peace within the glowing light of St. Patrick's Cathedral, when I am in New York. It was a healing experience then, and it is a healing experience now.

We want there to be more than this. We resonate to, and need the mystery of stained glass and majesty, the weight of the unbearable immensities beyond ourselves, and the sound of delicate silence.

1 *Lawrence E. Sullivan, director of Harvard University's Center for the Study of World Religions.*

2 *Thomas P. Kasulis, Ohio State University professor.*

- *The Second International Symposium on Science and Consciousness, William G. Braud, Greece, 3 Jan., 1992.*
- *Space and Time in the Modern Universe, Cambridge University Press, 1977.*
- *The Journal of Scientific Exploration, Stanford University, 1987.*
- *Engineering Anomalies Research, vol. 1, No. 1, p.21.*
- *Guilt is the Teacher, Love is the Lesson by John Borysenko, Warner Books, 1992.*
- *The Golden Bough by Sir James Frazier, MacMillan, 1992.*

# 6

## Ecology

I think you're beginning to know me by now. I don't deny I'm human and I don't like to dwell on my faults but what I have had to discuss with you up to this point is honest and well meaning, if a bit self serving. I hope you feel I'm someone you can trust into your home, and your mind. It's time to get to it. May I come in?

As I should be, I am a natural conservative. Some of you may think I am betraying my nature with the remarks to follow. If you do, think again. There are no convenient political pigeonholes any more. It's just that I take the Hippocratic Oath seriously. I care about the recovery and health of all my patients. My life and concerns revolve around the issues made important by the ill health I see around me, and I try not to let my training blind me to the biggest possible picture. Let's look at the forest, not the trees, for awhile.

Some hard rain is falling and **it's time we opened our eyes.**

Poll after poll, for decades, has shown a near 80 percent assent among the American people for efforts to clean up the environment, even if that might cost something! Obviously eighty percent of the American people do not have as much clout as the chemical industry. The gasoline in your car matters more than you do. This is known as "*democracy.*" Tell me I'm wrong. Please.

President Carter, one of the most moral of American presidents, whatever his faults, said, "*Pay attention, before it is too late, to one of the grimmest discoveries of the modern era.*" He was referring to hazardous waste, oil spills, and the general degradation of our environment.

Congress made a semi-effort to come up with a bill in response to President Carter's warning. The chemical lobby, and other assorted industries, brought counter pressure to bear upon Congress, so nothing happened. Meanwhile noxious poisons continue to pour into all the rivers and lakes of America. A good old country-river catfish can come close to killing you now.

The polluters are fond of pointing out that nature contains poisons too. I don't see this as much of an excuse. A balanced diet will keep natural poisons to a minimum and the body is likely to have evolved mechanisms to deal with them, which is probably not true of multiple body insults that come to us from an oil well or a coal mine.

President Ford had asked Congress for the same cleanup. The Environmental Protection Agency (EPA) spoke with forked tongue: "*Despite President Ford's position, the EPA must hold the line against any new spending programs, in order to fight inflation, and control the budget.*"

We have known for years that the EPA has allowed almost unlimited toxic substances into America's soil and foods, while Congress spends billions of dollars on weaponry, with no millions "*wasted*" on health. Now the most corrupt members of Congress want to do away with the EPA altogether. When you read the newspaper - **take notes**. There will be an election coming up somewhere soon.

I cannot understand why we can ignore this for generations (!), except to recognize a vast psychological denial at work. Obviously we don't want to know. We feel powerless. What can we do about it? Whenever we have a bad air day, we can smell what is pouring out of the smokestacks into the air. We are not the only nation that has gone into smokestack denial in this century. An old Yiddish saying is worth remembering in a larger context, "*Mir zeynen geknipt und gebinden.*" (We are all knotted and bound to one another.)

Industry called those of us who were concerned about toxic pollution "*chemophobics.*" They pointed to American know-how, and how in spite of kooks and tree huggers like us, our lives are made better through plastics and pesticides, chemicals, industrial solvents and automobiles - and besides they're doing all that can be done anyway.

The Mod Ag Biz is not taking action to grow healthier foods, cut the use of pesticides, phase out plans to irradiate foods, or carefully test and label genetically altered foods, as you might hope. No, in one case at least they are trying to get laws passed that will make it more *difficult* to advocate safer foods! Don't believe me? Read on.

We may remember the mess television personality Oprah Winfrey got herself into when she said some things about possible disease in American cattle. Major members of the American Farm Bureau Federation have been trying to get "*agricultural disparagement*" laws passed, so called "*Banana Bills*," that would require a "reasonable and reliable sound scientific basis" for any criticism.[1]

Sounds OK, but what would "*reasonable and reliable*" scientific evidence against a food polluter be? Our experience with the tobacco companies should convince us that it's unlikely that the Mod Ag Biz would accept even the best evidence if it threatened their bottom line. "*Strategic Lawsuit Against Public Participation*" (SLAPP) suits, nuisance suits used by corporations since the 1980's, are also a possibility. They are designed to bankrupt poorly funded nay-sayers, bell ringers, and "*eco-freaks*" with legal fees, not to establish the truth.

Banana Bills are on the books in 11 states, and are under consideration in 10 more, at this writing.

Florida farmers got a Banana bill passed which will force those convicted to pay three times the estimated dollar value of damage done to the Mod Ag Biz plaintiffs!

Monsanto, a bio-tech powerhouse, makes the growth hormone "recombinant bovine somatotropin" (rbST), which boosts milk production. They tried to keep other dairy producers from advertising that they do NOT (!) use rbST. In this case they lost. Can you believe this? Can you believe that the whole debate is totally without reference to any questions of right and wrong, - or truth? Of course my questions are rhetorical. We can all believe it these days.

I spoke out on the air about the level of malignant neglect, the toxicity, the abuses by industry. I spoke into a vacuum. We all know we live from, and off of, the soils and the seas of this planet. AIDS kills nowhere near as many people as does pollution.

How all encompassing our personal medical crisis has become! A Manichean battle between the Forces of Darkness and the Forces of Light has become part of everyone's nutritious breakfast. Ultimate questions follow us home every day. If we value our health and our lives, how dare we let our health become the losing half of a debate about profit!

Trees purify the atmosphere, produce oxygen, and absorb carbon dioxide. They are complementary to, and in fact part of, our lungs. Know it - trees are part of our lungs! What twisted and suicidal ignorance can lead the "*developed*" person in this "*developed country*" to chop his lungs out of the earth, or watch them die in the acid rain? Nowhere can I see the primary cause of our ill health more clearly symbolized! "*What can one say of the intimacy of intertwined branches, that know not each other?*" said Egberto Gismonti.

Somewhere along the road of life we may realize that there may be a universal truth, an ultimate reality, an ecology of the Earth. Everything seems to be interrelated, health and disease, healing and cure, thought and intuition. This is no less profoundly possible than what is there under the microscope.

Mathematics shows us how rapidly complexity multiplies when we increase the number of interconnected parts, and the recent news from the laboratories has all been of increasing subtlety, and increasing interconnections. Underlying our car payments and our daily frustrations lies a great mystery - and a great opportunity.

I know there are a lot of people in the world who say, "*I don't need you, I live an independent life.*" Their independence is like the independence of the roses in my rose garden. If we don't water them, if we don't till the soil, if we don't fertilize them, if the sun doesn't fall upon them in the right season at the right temperature, they will die.

Those of us who want to live alone on top of the mountain will discover that everywhere there are multiple issues we don't see or understand which nurture us (and we nurture them) and the connections between us all continue. There is a subtle conference going on, a symphony, of all that is within us and all that is without us.

Like it or not, we had better begin admitting that we are tied, cell by cell, to the outside world. Nothing in us exists alone and unconnected to the larger world. "*What happens to the earth happens to the sons of the earth,*" Chief Seattle may have said.

In a lifetime of reading, thought, and medical practice I am beginning to learn some hard spiritual lessons that many of you learned long ago. We are destroying the creativity of whatever we call the generative principle in the universe. Whether we call it God, or the operation of natural law, it is the force that "*drives the green fuse*", that denies chaos, and affirms life. It is this that we are attacking! It is for this reason, among others, that I recoil in horror at our current species destructions everywhere. **We are worshipping Satan!**

How dare we complain when Brazil burns its forests, while one of our own states (Alaska) is being deforested as quickly as possible, denuded of trees, *before we find out.* Who will share my outrage? Must we who care condemn ourselves to exile, to the periphery in our own decaying world?

Sooner or later all of us ask, "*Where am I? How did I get here? Why was I not consulted?*" We have all felt at one time or another like "*a stranger and afraid in a world we never made.*" Who is there to receive our complaints? Who is the jailer? We'd like a Suggestion Box, thank you.

I have spent a great deal of time in New Mexico and had the opportunity, in years past, to visit with some traditional Indian medical men. There was an old Indian called Lakota (the Sioux's own name for their tribe) who believed that Man's heart away from nature becomes hard. He believed that lack of respect for any growing, living, thing, sooner or later leads to lack of respect for ourselves. He needed therefore to keep in touch with nature. He believed that even the trees have conversations, not only with each other, but with humans who will listen.

Lakota pointed out to me that the White Man has one big problem: He never listens.

Go to a tree that has a lot of space around it where you can sit back quietly, silently face the direction of the sun, and spend a little while on each of your senses, seeing sunlight as it explodes on the leaves and dances through them. You will see ranges of remarkable colors from greens and browns to reds and oranges. See the flowers and shrubs, smelling, feeling, listening, to the hum of the insects. Or note the feelings, sensations, and spirit of Winter perhaps. The bare branches and clouds and passing birds. The whisper of wind. The melodies of the flowing stream.

Watch the deer, suddenly fearless, as you hold your breath. For the first time perhaps, feel the sun warm on your skin, the breezes through your hair, the scent of soil and grass. It is the most complex meditation we will ever experience.

If you spend time bringing each one of the senses into focus this way, away from the lies, dissonance and petroleums of the city, there is a contact you may never have had before. You sense a quality and creativity you may not believe is possible. It is a magic remedy which can open your senses, sharpen your focus, allow for a greater opportunity for intuition and creativity, and get you closer to the spiritual well of your existence.

In the book of Genesis, assembled prior to, and underlying, all three major western religions, it is stated, "*And the spirit of God moved upon the face of the waters.*" This serves to remind us of something important about all life on earth including ours.

Truly we could be said to be mobile, land dwelling, bags of primordial sea, our salt and mineral balances still not so very different. The smell of the ancient seas are about us, if I may break a minor taboo, when we are creating new life; and the deeper we delve into the secret inner structures of our cells, the more we see what we still have in common with the creatures of the sea.

We cannot live without water, our bodies are largely water, and the scientific study of our health must immerse itself in the chemistry and solubility of water. As the mystics have said, we are a fountain, which is never the same and ever the same. We are permeated with water. Water flows into and out of us while we live.

The resemblance of our body fluids to the seas of earth is not accidental. Our bodies work hard to create that ancient balance. If salt is too high, our body adds water, as much as four extra quarts, and pulls nutrients from our tissues, until our sea is in balance again. No wonder we get bloated and bleary when we eat too much salt.

What we do to the planet's water is being done to our bodies, and to all life. Obviously, questions of water purity must enter into our most intimate thoughts. There is a deep and profound evil in our world, and it is found everywhere, in every drop of water we drink. We must explore this evil, so that we will know what we must do.

As I was writing these remarks, a nightmare came together. Something was clawing at my mind. In my nightmare there was something looming in our future that is even worse than our dreams of flame, born at Hiroshima in 1945.

I dreamed that our destruction of the earth continues until our planet is a howling wilderness of struggling weeds, dust and mud, insects, and the few remaining small animals who bred fast enough to adapt; the seas dead except for toxic blooms of microorganisms. In my nightmare, mankind has become an eternal cripple living on a crippled earth!

But this is not why my dream was a nightmare. The worst is, that I see the crippled human race crowing in triumph! *That* is the nightmare!

The worst is that we laugh! We celebrate! We have won! We have conquered nature!

At long last we have succeeded in leaving the natural world. We are out of all ecological niches. At last we have learned what we mean to the earth. Mankind has prevailed, and we have become an abomination! A nightmare!

Yes, it was just a dream. We are slowly learning that our health is the health of the planet. We know how we should live so that we do not destroy the earth. Despite everything, I am optimistic, but within the next few years we must begin to act on our knowledge. If we do not, my nightmare will surely come to pass.

Until we act, we and our "*civilization*" will continue to drift into malaise, violence, poverty, ignorance, ecological devastation, and decline. We have not yet come close to facing the fact that the end of our present road is, *at best,* a new Dark Age. It's that serious!

**And surrounding our camp, out there under the moon, the lawyers are circling!**

Don't despair. If we beat with the pulse of the world, we will heal. We need to share the agony of the forests, of the mountains, of the sea. We need to ask the endangered life around us, our brothers and cousins in the world, for the courage we need. We need to let our love connect us with our creator, in gratitude. In the face of such a challenge, there can only be humility. If we learn this we will heal, and we may learn who we are at last.

The Indians tell of the hidden wisdom in the world which is available to everyone, even the White Man. The compassion the earth has for you, may well be discovered among the trees. The world will teach you. You will learn that you can't own it, until you find it within you. You will know how precious is the sky you can't purchase. Every tree is unique, every tiniest piece of land is different from every other, the earth is infinite!

With a rush of gratitude and holy dread we rediscover that we are, and always have been, a part of the earth. We need to explain to each other that surrounding ourselves with the world is not hypnotizing ourselves into numbness - **it is waking up!**

1 *Helen Cordes, The Utne Reader, Jan./Feb. 1996.*

- *The Environmental Working Group, (202) 667-6982.*

*Greatly expanded remarks about cancer are to be found in Chapter thirteen, and to a lesser extent in Chapter 17.*

# 7

## Mind, Body, and Healing

I'm going to take you behind the scenes in this chapter. I'm going to swarm all over the mind-body (psyche and soma - psychosomatic) question with you and look at it from a hundred directions. This is a big problem and we need to look at it from a lot of directions if healing is to have any meaning for us.

Before I begin I need to throw out a pile of ancient and destructive garbage. Egaz Moniz received the Nobel Prize in 1955 for his invention of the prefrontal lobotomy in 1936. I think I know why few objected to these insults to our brain. The reason is medieval and theological - and still part of our thinking! Our confusion destroys our clarity in our thinking about mind/body interactions.

Science has known for several hundred years that the mind is the brain thinking, the brain in operation, but very few of us believe it, even today. The word has not yet gotten around. We are stuck in the cave. Most of us assume the truth of the ancient idea of a split between the brain and the mind. When we ingest chemicals that affect the brain, we assume this has nothing to do with our mind. For this reason damage to the brain is not considered very important.

Religion, associated piffle about the soul as a rational thinking entity separate from our body, and ideas about reincarnation, play into this myth of the mind/brain split, as does all the "*New Age*" dithering about astral travel and "*out of body*" experiences.

In addition how many people ever use their mind for conscious thought? Someone who always reacts to the world in a mindless way is not going to miss, or defend, the possible loss of her "*mind.*" Too few of us care about, or remember, what we did two days ago. It didn't mean anything then and it certainly doesn't mean anything now. No matter what happens to our brain, we still expect to react in some mindless way to what happens to us, and to a great many people that is enough.

For these and allied reasons, we are not going to find ourselves immersed in massed anger when some new chemical or surgical assault on the brain is promulgated. Remember that fact when the surgeon wants to play with electrodes in our brain during our operation, or some new panacea for the pain of the world shows up on the shelves of our local drug store, or from our local pusher. Every pain we feel in our body is transmitted to our mind by our brain's outlying branches. Our mind is our brain which includes our entire body, so every drug we take also effects our mind, the so called brain barrier notwithstanding. I am not saying that chemical interventions in the brain are always wrong. In this world, unbearable tension, apprehension and dissension can easily get out of control.

We've heard too many horror stories about vital, intelligent, active, children who are considered "*hyperactive*" by the cold and grim authorities at school and are given chemical lobotomies so they will "*fit in.*" This is a class-bound political decision, not a medical one. One wonders what such monsters would think of a young Buddha or Jesus daring to question his teachers. Do we want young Einstein to "*fit in*?"

On the other hand, controlled studies have shown that "*a broad range of problems can benefit from psychological treatment*" in cases where the panic, anxiety, etc. that we feel, is irrational and not directly caused by outside reality. In those cases we could use some help. It is comforting to know that we can get it.

The problems referred to include phobias of many kinds which affect more than 10 percent of American adults, panic attacks which affect millions of Americans, anxiety with no identifiable cause, and the most common of all, depression.

Treatments include various forms of therapy such as cognitive therapy, interpersonal therapy, desensitizations, and meditation or relaxation. And of course the semi-scientific and expensively trendy pop therapies we all know and love. Various psychoactive drugs are available and for those who appreciate the goode olde medieval "*chop first and check later*" approach, there is still electroconvulsive therapy, which is just as horrible as it sounds. Your mind is affected and you won't like the side effects, if you should have a "*you*" left afterwards.

With all that safely out of the way let's talk of ships, and sails, and sealing wax, and cabbages and kings:

In 30 years in medicine, communicating with people who have complained and suffered, as well as listening to people who have phoned in to my radio shows, I have discovered that humans can occasionally regain their health simply by altering their point of view, their selection of emotions.

We don't select these things for ourselves - not anymore. The media get your attention with all those revolutions, terrorism, riots, coups, murders, kidnappings, sexual debasements, random violence, and economic exploitations on TV and in newspapers! That's what they are there for - to get our attention and to package us, in lumps of 1,000 for the sponsors. WE are what is sold on commercial television! These imposed belief systems have programmed out the good and the peaceful in us. The Establishment solution is more TV violence and more gun control. Why are we so surprised when disease hits us more often?

As I get further into this discussion of the effect the mind and body have on each other, I don't want you to forget that medicine is wonderful in its place. An antibiotic will probably still kill a staphylococcal bacterium. It would be ridiculous to remove oneself from the opportunity of using it. Mainstream "*allopathic*" medicine is extremely important and "*germs*" still sometimes kill. I wouldn't turn away from treatment that rapidly helps my problem, but I also want medicine that lets me mobilize my own healing mechanisms as well. We should take advantage of two systems for healing, one of which is outside ourselves, the other within.

Penicillin has given us the perception that Americans can be "*processed*" by an MD. This does not explain why we are so frightened by AIDS, why tuberculosis and malaria are haunting us again, and why we are overwhelmed by the occurrence of bacteria that have become resistant to our antibiotics. Strep throat is not usually fatal yet ordinary streptococci can become flesh eaters. We may be returning to square one, where antibiotics are useless, and bacteria still menace us.

Your attitude, actions, thought processes, responses, mythologies, etc. which are defined as good; will determine the chemistry and the natural immune system killer cell response, the good HDL, the heart rate, blood pressure, and the healed ulcer. "*Evil*" on the other hand dispenses to your body in the form of disease.

I don't want you to think that I am implying that, "*If I am ill, therefore I am bad,*" or "*I was bad therefore I became ill.*" I think guilt, stimulated by this kind of argument taken the wrong way, really destroys a person if they take it to heart. I don't see how it will help anybody heal.

On the other hand, to smoke or not to smoke is our decision. We choose to eat bacon or not. Some foods are the good parts of the life of our body. We could look to the moral issues of communal societal good versus evil as not different from the neural-physiological issues of good versus evil in the mind and body.

Thou shalt not pout and scream and taunt and rant and rave. Thou shalt not reach the point of violence, or thou wilt surely damage thyself. Anger expressed in certain ways shoots bullets.

We have all learned about coronaries. Those who are angry or hostile are the most nearly likely to bomb away their hots. A person acting "*apoplectic*" is a good candidate for apoplexy (a stroke). One of the best ways that we can begin to overcome our medical doom is to begin our threatened act of anger in a calm, quiet manner, forcing an artificial smile. We might try that tactic while listening to the evening news, standing in that steaming line at the market, or stuck in that traffic on the freeway. Start smiling like an idiot. Forget your dignity; it's your heart we are talking about!

Looking at that dumb rictus on your face in your rear view mirror or watching another's reaction, may actually make you laugh, and the volcanic mood is gone. You will discover that your mood actually follows the action, and the chemical fuse is pinched out. Then you can begin to do something physical to burn off the excess epinephrine (adrenalin) which can do a lot of damage otherwise. It may mean taking a walk, doing some exercise, or yoga. Is that so bad?

This is an interesting vein of thought. It illustrates vividly why we use meditation, yoga, Buddhism, and prayer. We're looking for utility, not truth. Morality may be a soothing victory for the interconnectedness of our white blood cell's immunity, amygdalin's sense of emotion, our ability to reason, and ultimately our good health.

I had a dentist come to see me from the same building as my office, with an ugly ear to ear rash on his face and on his hands. He said he'd been to umpteen dermatologists, he'd taken cortisone creams, and he was at his wits end. He wore a mask in the office but he was embarrassed to lean over in front of a patient because it showed through. His hands looked like they were going to infect the patient. He wore gloves which only made the rash worse. All the heavyweights were unable to help him. What should he do?

I said, "*Joe* (not his name), *why do you hate dentistry? And when are you going to change to something else? Maybe what you're failing to see is that you're not facial skin and finger hand skin at all. You're a body and a mind, and the mind has a secret you're ignoring. I would bet that you don't want to be a dentist.*"

He stood there, mouth open literally in shock, and said, "*No one ever asked me that question, but you know the truth is I hate it!*"

I told him that the reason he hates it is irrelevant. We need to walk through life doing what we enjoy. One way or another, that's where we have to make our living. "If you have to make your living hating every moment, I think you're going to have a whole lot more than just an eczematous rash." "*Thanks a lot,*" he said. "*Maybe you're right and maybe you're wrong. I can't just give up my living, but I'm sorry that I bothered you,*" and he turned to leave. I told him, "*You didn't bother me.*" He said, "*Well, you're bothering me,*" and he left unhappy.

In fact he was so unhappy with me for pointing this out that what he did do is forget to say hello to me in the elevator. On the other hand, about a year later around Christmas, I got a very nice case of wine. The note said, "*I hated your guts for pointing out what I didn't want to know because I didn't want to face it. I have sold my dental practice. My wife and I came up here to the Napa Valley, bought a near bankrupt vineyard. We work from dawn to dusk. We've never been happier or healthier. Rash gone. Thanks a million.*" (signed) Joe,"

We are beginning to learn what medicine can do, and what it cannot do. If you break your leg, medicine can help you, and meditation probably cannot, at least until the bone is set. A doctor can probably find your infected appendix, make a diagnosis, and get the antibiotic into you, a whole lot faster than your guru can. We can replace parts now, joints and hearts, transplant livers, fix hips. We have a million ways to cut you safely, and we are learning how to balance your hormones.

What we can't do is cure. We can't cure AIDS or any other virus disease. We can't cure chronic illness. We can't yet cure inflammatory illnesses like arthritis, and other auto-immune problems. **Cutting** or **Burning** or **Poisoning** a cancer is not curing anything. What we can't do is deal with mind-body related illness.

The amygdala we think, one of the oldest parts of our brain, is the mediator between our chemical intuitive emotions and our cognitive cerebrum, the rational, thinking, aware, portion of the brain. We recognize fear first as the felt emotion in the amygdala, and then as the brain's interpretation from the higher levels. People who are angry and fearful are more likely to have elevated cholesterol.

We need to look at other complementary forms of medicine as well, even at medicines relegated to limbo as quackery just a few short years ago. I believe in the value of well chosen alternatives, of the optional, of the complementary, when we are facing threatening illness. There is a place for acupuncture. There is a place for massages and herbals. There is a place for philosophy, a place for biofeedback, a place for body work, for oriental herbal medicine, homeopathy, even for color, flowers and aromas. There is a place for healing on a spiritual level. Is medicine a branch of religion - or vice versa? Does it matter? No one approach is enough.

A lady once came into my office and said, "*I've been to neurologists, psychiatrists, internists. They all think I'm nuts. I have migraine headaches that are impossible, almost daily now. I'm 44, and they won't go away. I had every pill known to help migraine sufferers. I've had all kinds of medications. I'm still sick! Can you help me?*" I sat with her and talked to her. I asked her all the questions. I asked her why she wanted her migraine.

"*That's a nasty question,*" she said. I assured her I hadn't intended it that way. I had intended it as an insightful question, because my perception, as a healer, was that she wanted her headache or she would have gotten rid of it. If all those pills didn't work, even pain pills, then she was fighting them. She started to cry.

She told me, "*When I was 12 my parents used to eat out every night because they did business that way, and I was alone constantly. I hated it. One night I had this terrible headache, and my mother told my dad to go off because, 'I don't want to leave her alone like this.' She was very kind to me that night. She put ice on my head. She was loving. I hadn't had that kind of attention in a long time.*"

"*I learned how to manipulate myself into the center of attention by having one of these terrible headaches. They even took me to doctors about it. Then the need receded when I was a teenager and I stopped having those headaches.*"

"*Now my husband never pays as much attention to me as when I have a headache, and my daughters only clean up the room and take care of the house when I have a headache. I use my headaches a lot. You know what, maybe I'm not ready to get rid of my headaches.*" She got up, paid my bill, and left.

I think she was inducing something, something she said she did not want. Perhaps we too can learn to avoid these addictions by coming into awareness.

About six months later I got a letter from her which said that she had found some better ways. "*I've decided life has to be lived differently. The more I try in these new ways, the less and fewer headaches I have. In fact this week I haven't had one, which is the first time since I was 21. I guess I thank both of us.*"

Stories like these don't happen with every patient of course. But when they do, they add depth and conviction to our basic understanding of medicine and the healers art.

When somebody becomes "*well*" when they're not "*supposed to*" this is called "*spontaneous remission from unknown causes.*" Rarely do we see that there might be some activity of our own body in bringing about such an event. This is the rarity the doctor tips his hat to, before turning away.

To affirm our life is to take responsibility for it. Will you do this? It means more than just whether or not we eat an egg; it is whether or not we cherish our cholesterol dreams. Our mental state determines our response to the world, psychologically and even physiologically. Like second-hand smoke, social abuse and violence affect non-participants.

Here are some of the symptoms of depression. Most of them are obvious but a few are not, so if things are not the way they should be with you, it might be a good idea to look the following list over:

- *1.) Persistent low, anxious, or "empty" feelings.*
- *2.) Decreased energy, fatigue, feeling "slowed down."*
- *3.) Loss in interest or pleasure in usual activities, including sex.*
- *4.) Insomnia, early-morning waking, oversleeping, or other sleep disturbances.*
- *5.) Appetite and weight changes (either loss or gain).*
- *6.) Feelings of hopelessness or pessimism.*
- *7.) Feelings of guilt, worthlessness, or helplessness.*
- *8.) Thoughts of death or suicide.*
- *9.) Difficulty concentrating, remembering, or making decisions.*
- *10.) Chronic aches or persistent bodily symptoms without physical origins.*

Sometimes things really are hopeless, but depression is never indicated. Please note that the objective situation (reality) may call for any or all of these feelings at various times. There is no criticism of you as a person implied in this list, and no matter what horrors have happened in real life, there may still be something you can do to lighten your load of troubles.

Anger, fear, grief, depression, sadness, and guilt are immune suppressers. They give the illness, the cancers, the coronaries, every opportunity to become worse. We survived before electricity and before penicillin.

You need to pay attention. Do you get enough sleep? Do you get the right nutrition? Do you have a healthy point of view and focus? Don't you need a nourishing diet rather than merely an adequate one? There are controversies about good diet, but I think we can bring it into clear and personal focus nevertheless.

Stress tears our bodies apart. At least 67 percent of all office visits represent stress-related circumstances and conditions. Physicians think of it as external pressure and forces, exerting outrageous and influential slings and arrows at us. DIS-ease!

Most popular magazines have informed us that the most common physical effects of stress are skin rashes, high blood pressure, heart failure, immune deficiency, cancer, virus and other infections, asthma, recurrent headaches, and most cardiovascular diseases.

Now a study out of Rockefeller University in New York finds that prolonged periods of stress kill memory-forming neurons in humans. Cortisol, a stress hormone released by the adrenals, may be responsible for our trouble remembering things as we age. There's no cure for the condition, so just remember don't worry, be happy. Sigh....

Our reaction to stress is not designed to increase our lifespan or keep us healthy. It is designed to help us escape from a lion. We respond, as our bodies evolved to respond millions of years ago, by biochemically adjusting us to either fight or flee. Do you think it is really such a good idea to allow our civilization to become so "*rational*" that we forget what we are?

We become victims of our ancient past. Several chemicals from the adrenal glands, including epinephrine, rush at us (that's what it feels like), causing all kinds of inappropriate or harmful body responses, including rapid heart rate, higher blood pressures, and higher blood sugars. We recognize the physical symptoms of stress within ourselves which triggers even more stress.

Stress has been linked with multiple skin disorders on a biochemical basis. Extra cortisol, extra epinephrine, and excess amounts of other hormones and neurotransmitters are released and linked when we are under stress. Nerve fibers release chemicals called neuropeptides under stress, which also lead inevitably to inflammation, aches, and pains. One of the neuropeptides, known poetically as Substance P, is especially likely to be potent in affecting one type of lymph cells, called "*map cells*." Once these cells are affected, they "*degranulate*" and spill out chemical activators of inflammation, and induce pain. Can psoriasis be far behind?

There's a direct relationship between psychological stress and significant suppression of our immune system. Stress seems to change our natural killer cells, reducing the proliferation of lymphocytes and prohibiting their ability to reproduce when stimulated to do so by invaders. These alterations play a major role in our susceptibility to any invasion which calls upon our immune system to be at its best.

Dr. Linus Pauling pointed out over 20 years ago that there is a very significant relationship between stress and the common cold. See Dr. Pauling's last interview later in this book (Chapter 16).

It is therefore quite clear that we must begin to learn stress reduction, which includes physical fitness and exercise according to our capacities, and psychological counseling whenever it seems necessary. Stress is reduced whenever we have a conversation with a real listener and a friend, and whenever we are authentic, face the situation, and make decisions as to what is changeable, what is not changeable, and how we choose to react to our reality.

A series of New Age tapes are available consisting of ocean sound and other sounds which are designed to reduce stress and tranquilize us. As music they belong on an elevator, but they might be useful to you if you have high blood pressure. Meditation, muscle control, and biofeedback also help.

Tibetan monks practice prodigious feats of visualization as part of their religion. Visualization, allied with prayer, has become vestigial in American thinking, thanks to TV and our world of no thought. Yet, we have oncologist after oncologist challenging their cancer patients to self help visualization and the use of their imagination. It may be as important, if not more so, than chemotherapy.

In guided imagery, you are asked to imagine yourself in some private, wonderful space where only you are present, lying on the beach as might be, where you feel yourself becoming less and less motivated to worry, and far more likely to become warm, loose, relaxed, and unhurried. One of the main self help medicines today is the relaxation response.

The trick is not to go out to a biofeedback practitioner once a week, but to do it daily at home in private and quiet. You can benefit, perhaps go sane, from going through the relaxation response at least 50 times a day for at least 15 seconds each time.

High blood pressure patients may want to experiment by joining a support group to undergo hour long meetings for a minimum of eight weeks of stress reduction. I'll bet at least three quarters of you are likely to lower your medication dosages.

Meditation is more than an Asian importation for trendy executives and aging hippies. In its most basic form, meditation is the silence in our stopping place, the space we clear for ourselves in our mind, the place where we can wake up, the place where we are able to confront and come to terms with the storm of change around us. Without that comforter, the storm without cannot be separated from the storm within, and we are left mindless and unhealthy in the face of chaos.

Maybe that's why meditation really is so important. We have to train ourselves out of all our addictions, to bring to focus the confusions we will not face, the obligations we think we have, the lack of our own authenticity and our own honesty, the perverse enslavement of our own thoughts.

We no longer look into the lion's maw. It's words, not teeth, that create our fear, words that create our anger, words that calm, produce love and healing, destroy political community. It was the words of God that created our world. It is our words that destroy it. A hungry lion is soon gone (or we are); he doesn't follow our every step, day in and day out, for a lifetime. We often hear that if you look into the hole long enough, the hole will look into you. We all know what that means.

We need to accept ourselves as we really are, live with authenticity, reduce our expectations, throw away our masks, and make sure all the lions are where they should be.

Too many of us are forced to learn about the body-mind connection from sales clerks in the health food store, and occasional writers like me who dare to talk about, and write about, a different kind of biomedical model.

As a medical resident I was able to demonstrate to my interns that I could take an 18 year old acute asthmatic admitted to the emergency service, and instead of administering the standard emergency intravenous drugs, could through conversation, reassurance, and the administration of saline placebo alone, work with his mind and body to the degree that I could bring that asthma sufferer to the point where he could go home.

I was teaching interns about the treatment of acute asthma. A young Latino was brought upstairs to the emergency floor with a "*red blanket emergency asthmatic attack.*" In order to quickly help a severe asthmatic attack we usually gave very tough drugs intravenously, theophyline, aminophylline, with possible cardiovascular risks.

Off the top of my head, intuitively (I'll get back to that below), I said to the intern who was racing to give him a 10 cc vial of aminophylline over a period of time, "*Hey wait. Let me show you that asthma can be talked out, it can be cured by conversation.*" They all looked at me. I'm sure they thought I was crazy.

"*Let me be crazy,*" I said. "*Get the aminophylline ready. Put it in a syringe. Keep it near you if I tell you I really need it. But first, let me give him a bottle of plain 5 percent dextrose and water intravenous (IV), and get the huge syringe ready that he's used to getting, 50 cc size. I will inject plain normal sterile saline, with a big needle, rather than medicine and I'm going to talk to this guy.*"

I sat down at his bedside, and I set up one arm with the IV and in the other arm I injected him with this big needle and it hurt, and I slowly, over the next few minutes, gave him the 50 cc that he knew from many times before was the treatment for his acute asthma.

I began talking to him in a slow suggestive hypnotherapist's voice. I told him what we're going to learn while we're doing this. I told him that we can get a much more rapid effect by learning how to breathe. I began discussing yoga methods of deep breathing, holding the breath and relaxing. We got into the relaxing mode. Relaxation induction is a lot like hypnotic induction: "*Let go. Loosen the muscles. Stop being afraid. You know this medicine works. You've had it before. We're going to be sure that it does work. In the meanwhile instead of keeping our mind on the medicine let's realize how we can keep our mind on ourselves and relax and change.*" The interns stood back and watched. Their jaws dropped. The room began to fill.

Within a matter of 10 minutes this man's asthma was fifty percent better. I said, "*Are you beginning now to get the effects of the medication?*" He replied, "*Well I don't have exactly the same feelings from the medication, but I'm beginning to feel much better.*" I told him, "*It's a newer brand with less side effects but it works very well. Let's just continue, but forget about the medicine.*"

The needle was now hurting his arm, which I willfully kept there. I injected the saline slower and slower while I talked with him. In half an hour I talked this man, age 18, totally out of a red blanket emergency asthmatic attack, on sterile saline!

I asked myself then, and I have asked myself many times since, how is it that no one taught me this? How is it that it's not in the books? How is it that placebo effects are genuine? How is it that the doctor is in fact part of the medicine? How much of a role do I play other than simply sticking my patient with "*aminophylline*?" The mind-body connection was totally at work here.

**How much of established medicine is placebo?**

I have a feeling that a nurturing relationship between doctor and patient, healer and healee, needs to be the hard core center of a lot of what we do, but thanks to modern politics, that is going to be ignored and forgotten. There is nothing in any HMO that allows for "*off the top of my head, intuitive*" medicine as I described it above in regard to the young asthmatic. Anything that departs from the clinically and philosophically sterile in medicine detracts from the scientific bottom line. Once the "*bottom line*" was the health and well-being of the patient. No more.

If I were to seriously advocate practicing medicine "*off the top of my head, intuitively,*" I would be justifiably up for instant peer review by a committee of MDs at best, and on the carpet (thick and luxurious) in front of a committee of MBAs at worst, yet how can the art of medicine advance with no caring, no imagination, no intuition, no patient/doctor dialectic? So many "*health professionals*" today are ready to leave it all to the computers, and the thick books of standard practices.

Now is a good time to talk of placebos. An undeniable physical effect from medical placebos (sugar pills) illustrates the fact that, "*Patients can sometimes benefit from a thorough medical evaluation, a diagnosis and a plausible plan of treatment whether medication is given or not, Patients enjoy the enthusiasm, effort, commitment and respect of their doctors and nurses. These factors are not incidental to the healing process.*" They provide an important clue as to why placebos work.

Somewhere I read that, "*The healing environment is a powerful antidote for illness. The decision to seek medical assistance restores some sense of control. The symbols and rituals of healing - the doctor's office, the stethoscope, the physical examination - offer reassurance. An explanation for the illness, no matter how scientifically tentative, and a prognosis, when favorable, reduce fear. Physicians can incorporate aspects of the placebo effect, in ways that are both medically and ethically sound, to make accepted medicines more effective.*"

This must be carefully done of course. I feel a bit ambiguous about anything that can be said to be fooling the patient, no matter how well intended. Perhaps amused candor is the best stance toward placebos.

All we can say with any degree of certainty is that healing is not caused by healers, whether they come to us with stethoscope and medical degree, acupuncture needles, homeopathic remedies, the cachet of thousands of years of tradition immersed in ancient cultures, feathers and smokes and drums, robes and incense and cross, germicides of all kinds, or even "*modern*" (and untried) alternative therapies.

Yet when we have specified what healing is not, we still are left with its mystery. Somehow it is involved in love, compassion, empathy, caring. Those who must heal alone are in grave danger. Healers of all cultures and all ages have talked of the truth of this. We are all witnesses to forces beyond our control.

We ignore the patient with rheumatoid arthritis who always knows when stress has made the situation worse, causal "*germs*" notwithstanding. Many others might find help in mediating these classic ailments: ileitis, ulcerative colitis, and diarrheas, despite the nominal cause; in meditation, biofeedback, hypnotherapy, psychotherapy, or a change in life style.

More heart attacks happen on Monday morning from 9 to 11 AM than at any other time! Studies have shown that people who see the world as an angry place (which it certainly is) have nearly six times the likelihood of dying too soon from an acute heart attack than do people who somehow manage to do what? Fool themselves? Rise above it all? Rage is a serious disorder. It releases those fight-or-flight chemicals which squeeze blood vessels in your heart muscles, causing a pain much like angina. Rage tampers with your entire human physiology. It allows cancer cells to happen by the abundant rise of free-radical molecules. Rage raises blood pressure as well as speeding the heart rate. The scene for disaster is set.

Japanese doctors see a variety of illnesses as mind catalyzed. They call some diseases "*autonomic nervous system upset.*" How can the autonomic system be said to be balanced under rapid heart rate, cold skin, wide eyed fear, and tension? A medicine like Valium is a manager of symptoms. There is no true curative meaning to America's multi-million dollar pain killer market. We might think of Valium or its counterparts as just "*dry alcohol.*"

Our neurotransmitters, including endorphins in our brain, are the carriers of our feelings. I don't think anybody would deny that the human neuropeptides, so far identified, link the immune system, the glands, the brain, the psychology and physiology of the body, but nobody puts the pieces together. We are in fact, not only what we eat, but also the way we philosophize, the thought before the act, the spirit on the wing, the way we behave, both singly and collectively.

I have often discussed these matters with physicians. They have felt uncomfortable, and replied that if the body is so smart, the DNA so well trained, and the immune system so perfect, and the healing system is so "go," *why do people get sick?*

The answer of course is that we injure those systems. We injure them with uncontrolled thoughts, smoke and pollutants in everything we touch or eat, the ultraviolet light that causes cataracts, the small molecule cholesterols (LDL) in our diet, the free radicals that we induce in our bodies, our lack of physical fitness.

In my medical programs on radio I talked of the art of living. The program director sometimes told me I was sermonizing. My answer had to be, "*You bet I'm sermonizing! Health is not merely butter, eggs, and vitamin C. Living healthfully is as much art as the paintings of Picasso or Rembrandt.*" The masterpiece that makes us human is the ability ultimately to learn to live to the point.

We must walk together or we all walk in darkness. We cannot be healthy alone. We need to make a different kind of choice.

We all have the need, the imperative, and the wonderful opportunity to become the artist and creator of our own lives and we don't let ourselves know it.

Often without our own knowledge, we act on our emotions in a million subtle ways that turn our days dark, sour our friendships, deaden our emotions and our creativity, distort our vision, skew our decisions and our votes, and begin to change the chemical balances in our immune system, or our arteries, in unhealthy ways. Fear - it's not just for breakfast anymore! Our T-cells know!

With aimless doing alone, we can perform something awful. Wrapped into the skeleton of doing has to be the flesh of feeling and attitude. The Buddhists call it right aspiration. Jewish wisdom calls it right feeling. Of course we don't know what truth is, but are we searching for it? How many of us will admit that we know, have sought, dare find, the truth of ourselves?

When we find a gun in our face in that dark parking lot, as has happened to me, we have a reason to walk in fear through our lives. The absolute conviction that comes with forcefully presented reality can warn us, but it also can distort us, and we must dance on the surface of these all too easily acted-out prophesies, so that the world we live in is ours, and not constructed of verbal poison from some street punk.

Our problem is not gun control, it is fury. Look at the thousands of people driving around you on the highway, front, back, beside you, and see nothing but hostility. Think of this when you stand in line somewhere, or talk to someone. Anger is a killer. National anger, bottled up, can lead to all the horrors of this past insane century.

I think that we're in a state of overload. Pressures are everywhere. Our culture has ceased to be something that everyone can participate in. When only an elite can control what's going on, how can we hope to continue our democracy, or protect our health? Inevitably, and always, we come to the political aspect of health don't we?

"*What the caterpillar calls a catastrophe and the end of the world, the master calls a butterfly*," is an ancient Chinese saying.

Jishnu (Jesus) Krishnamurti said, "*We must acknowledge that we are the anger, that we are the violence. If we can stay with this perception long enough, the whole structure of thought and feeling will collapse like a house of cards. We will no longer sense the thinking part of the mind as a separate entity that can comprehend, and perhaps control, the emotional part. Instead, we will see the emergence of a different kind of mind, in which thought and feeling, the observer and the observed, are one.*"

We have reached the point in America where our private insecurities, depressions, fears, guilts, and angers, fanned by the media, may lead us to vote for "*an end to confusion*" on a national level. Beware! Resolution of fear and doubt can be politically dangerous! "*No more doubt,*" they will tell us! "*Decisive action!*" Deadly action! The Triumph of Our Wills! Let us not forget that there is no healing in final solutions!

If we have a clear awareness of a situation, then coping will become more and more precise. We need to develop clarity and focus, I call it "*living to the point*," in order to banish our illusions. Some people call this clarity "*consciousness*." The Buddhists call it mindfulness. We must wake up from our profound sleep!

Why do we have so much time for fear and anger, for malice, for greed, and so little time for love, as the night approaches?

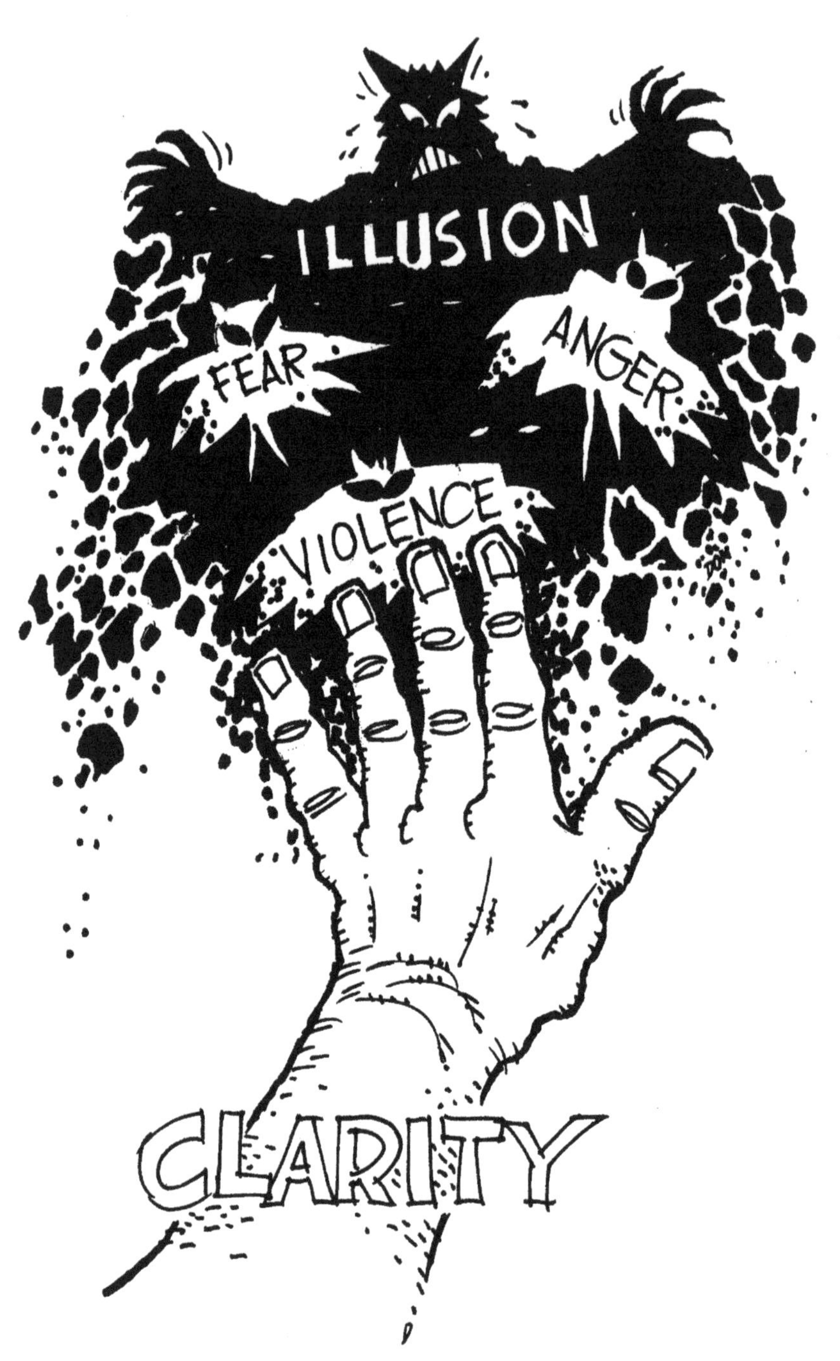
ILLUSION
FEAR
ANGER
VIOLENCE
CLARITY

# 8

# Young and Old

## Part 1: Young

I remember when I took my first boy for his first haircut when he was about three years old. Sitting in the barber's chair he began to cry. I said, "*Hey, hey, hey! Big boys don't cry.*" That marvelous barber said, "*Hey, hey, hey! Are you ever wrong! Why are you teaching him something as negative as that? It's reasonable for him to cry.*

"*He's a little kid in a big chair, and a big mirror, and big men are standing over him, and I have a shining instrument of destruction in my hand, and I'm coming at him, and he doesn't know why or how, or what's going to happen! As far as him being brave and courageous, he'll get around to war soon enough!*" I hope that man is still cutting little kids hair. That was a prince among barbers! His advice may save my boy's life 50 years down the line.

Abraham J. Heschel said, "*Let the young remember that there is a meaning beyond the absurdity. Let them be sure that every deed counts, that every word has power, and that we all can do our share to heal the world, in spite of all the absurdities. Above all, let them remember to build a life as if it were a work of art.*"

For instance, nothing illustrates the bankruptcy of commercial television more than children's programming. The Corporation for Public Broadcasting does a good job on the whole. Even The Great Purple One and those Creepy Tubbies are probably harmless, but the CPB can't make up for the vast wasteland on every other channel.

Did you know that fear of crime in the streets makes your children fat? McLuhan was right - the medium is the message! Even as we complain about the violence on TV, we use TV as our prime baby sitter. All those hours in front of the boob tube have a physical as well as an emotional and moral effect on our children. A study of over 4000 children showed that the more time they spent in front of the tube shirking exercise, the fatter they tend to be. Public health experts remind us that childhood obesity is a good predictor of adult weight problems. The study also documents that black and Latino children spend much more time in front of TV than do Anglos. Not hard to understand when mom or dad don't dare let the kids play outside. We protect their bodies at the expense of their minds.

Children need models much more than they need critics. Look at the models they've got!

In spite of everything, our children usually turn out well, and for that we should give thanks. They are also clear eyed. They are facing some horrifying lessons about the world we have made for them. We should not be surprised at their anger, fear, and tension. We must do what we can for our children, for we love them. We know the medical price they will pay. Dare we think of the political price?

The National Health Child Survey of 3000 elementary school children discovered recently that the lads and lasses knew what good nutrition was, they just ignored it. More than half of them had eaten no fruit or vegetables, or just one, on the previous day.

I remember those horror stories that my oldest son used to bring back from his "*progressive*" grade school. The little blighters were learning "*sharing*", and for almost a year, the boy learned all about bad nutrition, as he threw away the healthy veggies we had prepared and "*shared*" heavy doses of nitrates, fried cholesterol patties, plastic cheese with mayonnaise, a vegetable called ketchup, and caffeine laden pop, with the other kids.

Kid's diets are more important than the profit and loss statements of the national school food service corporations. When will telling children to eat the proper balanced meal, actually match what we prepare for them in school? That is the last argument that a Congressperson will understand. National priorities determine what we "*can afford.*"

No one gets alarmed enough to act regarding the massive and steady advertisements for sugar loaded cereals and fat, salt, and nitrate laden junk food aimed, on the Saturday morning TV wasteland, straight at the bodies of our children.

In the age range 11 to 18, girls in one study ate more than twice the protein and sodium recommended in government guidelines and more than one and a half times the phosphorus. Children are usually served a magnesium deficient diet. Excesses and deficiencies like this can increase the risk, small to be sure at this age, of cancer, hypertension, and osteoporosis in girls and young women.

Things aren't getting any better. There are several different packs of convenient "*poison-lite*" lunches being marketed these days so you don't have to bother to prepare your kid's lunch.

We were reminded recently of dumb ways to save tax money, and of all of them, not feeding poor pregnant women and their kids is the dumbest. We tell ourselves that we are the most advanced and civilized of the globe's inhabitants, while 20 percent of America's children are undernourished, and hundreds of thousands are homeless.

We have become, says the 1991 Senate Judiciary Committee report, "*the most violent and self destructive nation on earth, with a new breed on the street of criminally intense people, totally void of conscience, a breed likened to a mutant human animal growing more rapidly than any virus, deranged too often by drugs or the joy of violence, now capable of the most heinous, despicable, bestial acts, with a characteristic lack of remorse and absolutely no sense of wrong, and a gross, immediate, and terrifying total disregard for human life!*" How do I know this is true? Television showed me.

Our teenager's greatest challenge is trying to find out what good behavior is, without being able to see any of it. Doctors may, in fact, be the worst parents among us. They tend to control everything and fail to understand the nature and value of unconditional love. Childhood is too often defined as "*when you learn to follow all the rules.*"

***We are the victims of a relatively contemptible congressional array of blowhards, promising anything to anybody with enough money to get them re-elected, with about as much moral fiber as soggy rice flakes. All of us are the victims of a monstrous lack of leadership, a monstrous social incompetence, a monstrous indifference, and an***

***unclear middle class that doesn't know enough any more even to get angry, but just wants to know if it's OK to eat nonfat yogurt.***

A lack of inexpensive micro-nutrients for children helps explain why so many extra child deaths occur in less developed countries. A study in Sazawal showed that children with often fatal diarrhea improved with a zinc supplement of 20 mg a day. Indigent African American Women on 25 mg of zinc a day had far more healthy babies in another study. In Chile the same result was found with only 3 mg of zinc a day. We know that supplemental vitamin A (beta carotene would be better) reduces death from severe measles in children. UNICEF recommends vitamin A for children in developing countries at the time they are immunized against measles in their first year.

**Part 2: Old**

Some of my patients thought they were sinking into senility because they couldn't add a few simple numbers together (usually they were adding up my bill). They forgot that if you don't do something long enough, you'll forget how to do it. Our years of physical overload, and lack of attention to our health, show in every test our doctor makes.

Remember what we thought of people our age when we were a kid? Now the stairs are getting higher, the tennis courts bigger, the muscles sorer. Do you think it's possible the years have crept up on us too? Is it time to do what needs doing, and stop what needs stopping, and begin preparing to live forever?

The mind does not stop at the neck! We must not forget that we are our bodies! The nerves in our brain are connected to every organ in our bodies, and who is to say that some of our mind does not reside in our liver, or our little toe?

We have been abusing our bodies, and allowing our immune systems to lower the body's defenses. Our minds have lived through every moment of this. We have not noticed what we are eating, how we are moving and what we are breathing, or our spiritual needs, and how our angers and fears affect us.

I tell people, who come to me with these comments, that healing is built into our bodies, no matter what our age. We could blame our ancestors and our age for our illnesses and our slide down that hill, but I'll bet we have chosen to be where we are. Cigarettes, booze, legal and illegal drugs, fat in everything we eat, stress, attitudes, lack of exercise, may be the cause for our discontents. I want you to know that we can also choose a quality longevity!

Hidden under that layer of lard, flabby muscle, and inertia, can be a fit and more youthful person. Our body is not as old as our choices have made us think it is.

The old learn to think of themselves as being in the "*twilight of their lives*," as "*senior citizens*" in their "*golden years*." This crap demoralizes old people, who learn to play roles spelled out for them by the needs of television advertising, and the misunderstandings of youth. Beware of the self-fulfilling prophecy. It's true that young people are more physically capable and active, but they're not more intelligent or wise. The spiritual and mental attributes of the old can add wisdom, seasoned creativity, and even humor, to our culture's balance.

It's true that short term memory tends to get a little fuzzy later in life, so that someone 70 years old would need to keep in mind that they must subtract the last 10 minutes from their 70 years in any comparison with someone 25 years old.

There is an art to forgetting. What we remember and recall best is what we probably ought to have forgotten. I think it was Benjamin Disraeli, Prime Minister of Great Britain, who said that, "*It's Man's characteristic to suffer, and thankfully his fortune to forget. To remember much is not necessarily to be wise.*"

Only a small number of brain cells disappear because of aging. A study at the Salk Institute in La Jolla demonstrated that mental challenge could dramatically increase the number of cells in the hippocampus of laboratory animals. "*Intellectual stimulation during life's later years can still influence the architecture of your brain,*" says Fred Gage. Humans can grow new brain cells in later life. It is possible for the brain to renew itself by growing new connections.

And, be sure to remember, learning is one of the greatest pleasures of life.

The only proven causes of brain deterioration, aside from certain well described diseases and conditions such as Alzheimer's disease, endocrine imbalances, anemia, diabetes, malnutrition, chronic infections, lung disease, tumors, drug reactions, and severe vitamin deficiencies, are chemical abuse from alcohol or other mood altering drugs, and lack of use.

There is also an art to using time. Inscribed on an ancient sun dial is, "*Time WAS is past. Thou canst it not recall. Time IS thou hast. Employ thy portion small. Time FUTURE is not. And may never be. Time PRESENT is the only time for thee.*"

As we grow older, and mentally stronger, we can bring happiness to those around us. We can give out more, and take in less, love more, and we may also begin to find some of the meanings we have been looking for, and learn how to share all this with others as well.

I have often quoted an old saying, "*May you die young, at a very old age.*" Another saying comes to mind, "*It's not how old you are but how you are old.*" I don't think that we should go through life "*face lifting our age.*" There is something strange about people who live a 35 year youth, a 45 year middle age complete with hair dye and plastic surgery toward the end, and then move out of town to hide a very short old age, and death. We should admire or at least respect our wrinkles. We earned them. They attest to what should be the fine wine of our life.

When I was nine years old my father and I had dinner with the attorney Louis Nizer, and then never saw him again. He became very big and very famous. If you wanted him, you put down a $250,000 corporate retainer to start and that was non-inflated money. When I became an attorney myself, I went to a judges dinner and Nizer was there. I was in my 40's by then.

I walked over to him and said, "*Mr. Nizer, I'd like to congratulate you on your last book. Thank you for the speech you made tonight. It was brilliant. My name is Gershon . . .* " Before I could finish, Nizer said, "*Wait a minute. You're Gershon! You're telling me that I am a very old man! That's not true. I've been a very young man for a very long time. Gershon Lesser, how are you?*" He was in his 70's at the time, with his remarkable memory still intact.

We know that creative contributions from everyone really are going to be necessary in the tough times ahead. I view our elders as worthy to face the challenge of building a newer, saner, and more humane America. They still remember the dream.

I have an old photograph of my great grandma, taken shortly before her death, holding a baby in her arms. The baby was me. She must have been born about 1850. When my great grandma was a little girl, the Revolutionary War (not the Civil War!) veterans were still in their 80's. It hasn't been long enough for all of us to entirely forget the American dream.

Wrinkles are not the occasion for a discrete injection of some fatal poison, or even a $20,000 dollar face lift, but a hearty invitation to battle! What do you think all those years were for? Now you're ready, dad and mom. We need you! We need the elders of our tribe! Where else could wisdom possibly reside?

My father used to quote Newton, "*If I have seen farther than others it is by standing on the shoulders of giants*" while we, in our turn, have shrugged, thereby sentencing the young to reinvent the wheel.

The older population is growing but the internal medicine training programs still prepare trainees or internists to care for young vigorous patients with very limited chronic illness. It's a one dimensional disease-specific or organ-specific approach. Geriatric education is now almost nil and getting worse. If they don't break the traditional barriers of the residency training program, then geriatrically trained doctors won't exist. And destroying the program to save money is no solution.

What then is our standard to be? The debates about Medicare have made it quite obvious that to many in America, being old is a liability to the State.

The physician is supposed to be a healer. Can this be reconciled with helping the patient to die? If "*your right to die*" is not reviewed with serious care and concern by you and your peers, it may soon become your patriotic duty to die! Is murder to become a new medical specialty which we need to develop; tough doctors to handle that tough decision? Where does a doctor who is not trying to heal, fit? Dr. Linda Emanuel, vice president for ethics standards of the

AMA said, "*We do not have a right to die, but we do have a right to be free of unwanted intervention.*"

Medicine having become a business, now listed on the stock market, is less and less philosophic, less and less moral, less and less a vocation, and much more competitive and part of the economy. What is the economic potential of euthanasia?

I cannot justify turning over a life and death decision to someone who may have an agenda, as for example a hospital filled with richer patients, younger ones, requiring less attention.

Pope John Paul II in the encyclical, Evangelium Vitae, stated that the health profession has a "*unique responsibility to be guardians and servants of human life. The health profession is meant to be an impassioned and unflinching affirmation of life. True compassion leads to sharing another's pain. It does not kill the person whose suffering we cannot bear.*" He warned scientists not to become "*manipulators of life*" or "*agents of death.*"

I, as a lawyer, as well as a physician, am aware of the complexities of this issue. Whether someone who is terminally doped to the gills in order to kill pain is still human, is a question I am willing to debate, and I suspect that a brain dead body is a dead body, whether its heart still beats or not, but active action leading to the death of a living human being I will not tolerate or debate.

Albert Camus wrote, "*Suicide is the only truly serious philosophical problem.*" If life isn't worth living, then why bother. If life carries its own validation in the simple living of it, why ask. If life is sacred, then it's out of our hands.

Many of you, chances are, still nourish the stereotype of an older person as a seriously disabled, lonely, solitary human, bent over and drooling, going quivering and without dignity into that good night.

A better stereotype, if you must have one, might be a Golda Meir as premier of Israel, a Linus Pauling in his 90's running his own institute and doing it well until the day of his death. Remember Grandma Moses, who took up painting in her 80's, and became world renowned? Creativity didn't seem in short supply for any of these old and marvelous people.

I remember the artist who painted unflinching clear eyed nude self portraits in her old age. The marvelous guts and gall of it! Pablo Casals, the great cellist, never retired. Neither did guitarist Andres

Segovia. Pablo Picasso was painting and fathering children until his extreme old age.

It is an assumption of the young that the old have lived their life and have no further value, as though human life were a commercial transaction with a sliding scale depending upon age, beauty, wealth, lobbyists, and pressure groups. Who dares judge the creative need in another's breast? Have we become so corrupt as to toss the opera Falstaff into the trash because Verdi was over 70 when he wrote it?

Should we have destroyed the young sculptor before he carved his David because he was gay? Can we deny the same man, 40 years later, painfully climbing the scaffolds in the Sistine chapel day after day to dedicate the burning flame of his genius to the glory of God? What are we thinking? What have we done to ourselves?

We don't think of people like this, as we talk about the sudden political need in America to set limits for a rapidly aging population. The real lack, the critical resource we are running short of, is lovingkindness (compassion).

I once wrote a book titled "*Growing Younger*," and there are magazines about longevity (*Longevity* for instance), yet we have a perception and a mythology that the power of the intellect and the creativity of the soul are only in 30 year olds, when in reality if you look at the age of the world's greatest accomplishments they were often developed like fine champagnes and mature wines that aged well. Frank Lloyd Wright's masterpiece *Falling Water* was designed and built when everyone thought his career was over! His reasoned answer to the question of the best architect's approach to the problems of Los Angeles came when he was in his late 80's. The answer by the way was "Evacuate."

The political dimension of health must be faced. Considerable evidence exists that critical care is being rationed in the United States, that not all care expected to be beneficial is available to all patients who want it. It's an everyday occurrence in most hospitals. The evidence is substantial, and the current rationing is highly unfair.

A group of "*social planners*," a title which makes me cringe, have set down their own malignant perception of old age, as a time of solitude, unproductivity, and social and fiscal waste. They have, in fact, as a matter of "*principle*" and policy, rejected old age as a luxury this country can't afford. No half civilized people could possible come to this conclusion. I am amazed and appalled.

Look head on at the new morality being sold today. It's not just the cost. They seem to think it is somehow wrong to keep people alive too long! None of today's "*social planners*" are talking of life enhancement, of the dignity of old age, and a challenge to increase its quality, or of any moral aspect of our need to protect our parents and grandparents from the fiscal impoverishment of disease. They seem to have no place for the nature and meaning of human life, as they deny old age any essential integrity!

Entitlements like Social Security and Medicare, that involve all Americans, sooner or later look mighty tempting to the politicians in Cashington, D.C. Creative bookkeeping can do wonders when you're trying to hide some pork and get ready for the next election. All they have to do is shout "*Giveaway!*" and the voters salivate on cue.

We must get medical costs under control. No argument. But must we do it the Cashington way with a little profit for everyone and no change of priorities? If you're rich enough to afford a lobbyist, Congress has something for you.

I don't suppose you've heard lately that Medicare is not a government handout but is paid for solely by the insured? You may not have imagined the abuse and misuse, the outright theft and waste that are there under the surface of the health care "*crisis*." A Lot of Medicare money is incorporated into debt and tax accounting when it was supposed to be sequestered for health care use only.

Your "*representatives*" make it sound like Medicare is a giveaway when the fact is that if your private money had been invested in a businesslike manner, and only paid out for claims, there would have been about 250 million dollars profit last year. The fact is Medicare never really had a loss, nor would it have a loss in the future, if the money had not, and was not, being misused. It was profitable right from the start before Congress got its hands on it.

The same thing is true of Social Security. I don't expect our government to be honest with us, or honor its promise (!) for a comfortable retirement for all working Americans, but it stings when money intended for Social Security is robbed to pay for Cape Canaveral, Saudi Arabia, and Mexican pesos. Remember that it was

Joseph Goebels, Hitler's propaganda minister, who said that a lie repeated often enough and loud enough will be believed.

Look as hard as you want and you won't find a federal account where Medicare, or Social Security money is paid in, or is collecting any interest. Our promises got mingled with general federal funds for anything government wants it for. Meanwhile it's real easy to make us feel guilty. Sorry Senator, I don't think I'm ready to take the blame for this one!

The "*social planners*" have determined what is the determinant of the availability of health care. When I think of any social planner telling me that my mother is just too expensive I blow a little smoke out of my ears. "*This is still the United States of America!*" as indignant Americans used to say when I was young.

We must not forget that from a moral point of view, our age is as much an accident as our race, or our gender. It is a biological fact, and must not become a part of any program of purification, or cleansing, lest we join the other monsters of the last century - the century of the damned.

Death I promise you will still condition all of our lives, but it is not for anyone to determine how long it is rightful for us to live, or to receive healing care. This is not legitimate controversy, this is evil!

People of any age can lose so much of their zest for life that they are actually suffering sensory deprivation. If you can't stand to read the newspaper or watch TV, try one of those video games your kids (or grandkids) play, until you get good at it. Or buy one secretly for yourself. Keep up with your world. Eavesdrop on the young without censure.

Discuss their classes with your children or grandchildren, and actually listen to what they say. I tried that, and the best conversations I ever had in my life resulted. Try listening to your mate the same way. You don't have to be the family expert every moment. One of the causes of our anger is the knowledge that we're out of touch.

I must say to the older person, "*Maximize your advantages! Share in your righteous portion of the social pie. Seek to prolong your precious life in every way. Never, never, never, never give way to those who will succeed you, until you must.*" Teach the world, you elders, that in the collective wisdom of your years, you have indeed found your sense of place and purpose.

I know. In spite of the truth of all of this, we never forget that we are nearing the end, and everyone is afraid of dying. It is our greatest fear. It is the defining proof of human consciousness.

Let me share a parable about death with you - and a frightening question: Last night, it must have been around 2 or 3 AM, I woke with agony clutching my chest. In the seconds remaining, as I fell back dying, I prayed for more time. I have loved ones who need me, I have uncompleted tasks, I need more time to share my love with the world. In my parable I prayed for the time to get into good health, and finally to stick to my diet, and begin exercising. Then my heart stopped and I slipped into the eternal nothingness of death.

But somehow our prayer is always answered. A miracle occurred this morning. We woke up from death. Now we stand, immersed in miracle, once again alive. And I ask all of us that terrifying question:

"*Now what do we do?*"

# 9

## Or Are You Just Glad To See Me?

There's always room for another sex book at the bookstore. There are shelves full, libraries full, vast collapsing drifts and windrows of sex books blowing in the wind, not to speak of the tapes and net addresses, and movies, and magazines. You don't think I am going to try to compete with all that in this chapter do you? It might be fun to try - but no.

The chapter title comes from that generous spirited and affectionate comment by actress Mae West: "*Is that a gun in your pocket or are you just glad to see me?*" Let us cherish our physicality, our fumblings and mistakes, our ambition, our humanity. Let us fuck the whole earth and let the whole earth fuck us back! **I am talking about love.**

When we are young we can fool ourselves so easily as we tear the world apart verbally. We like to talk and joke about sex. At other times we talk of true love. We also remember every first time. We get used to the excitement and amazement of it all, have our children, get bored, and start worrying about last times.

Sex is a good way to burn calories pleasurably. It decreases a man's chance of getting cancer of the prostate. It can induce relaxation and calm in everyone, and vastly increase our chances for human touch, caring, and intimacy. As we get older we claim to get better. We also get slower. That's OK - We also get more grateful.

That's how a chapter about love (sex) should sound. If we are lucky, and if we retain some of our joy and youth, and if we stay open to possibilities, then we may one day learn that life is all one thing, and if we are truly lucky we will learn that this one thing is the universe. Sex is love, is our connection to everything, is our body complete and all of our mind and our holiest connections to God.

This is the true and real thing. All of our insecurities and boredom and temptation are the true and real thing also.

Everything that can be said about the philosophy of sex, the mechanics of sex, the results of sex, the morals of sex, sex and the law, sex and religion, the pathologies of sex, the diseases of sex, the doing of sex, sex and the universe, and the encouragement or discouragement of sex, has been, and is constantly being, said. Please see the appropriate sex manual, a good therapist, the proper video, or even an understanding minister or rabbi, for your answers. A satisfying sex life is part of good health.

As you've probably heard, the single most important sex organ is the brain. It deals well with the right mood, candles, unrushed time and spontaneity, and down by the shore an orchestra's playing! Finally you should keep in mind that your violence box (your TV) can get you in the wrong mood real quick. The late night talk shows don't turn many people on. It might be a good idea to move the television out of the bedroom, and into the garage where it belongs, unless you have something special in the way of video tapes.

# 10

## The Boob Tube

As long as the subject came up, I guess we should talk about television.

We let television tell us who we are and what we should do. Our definition of health is what we see, or don't see, on television. We judge our diets, exercise, and moral state, by the images on our TV. It's clear that commercial considerations determine our reality. There's no longer any objective test of our humanity.

Reality, we are taught by television, is the androgynous adolescent wet dream floating diaphanously through the pavilions of some never never land half way between violence and perversion. How we actually feel is not persuasive until validated by TV. Our unique personal optimum has lost its meaning. Our endurance, our wisdom, our feeling of being at home in our body whatever its age, no longer signify. After a great deal of thought over a period of many years I cannot escape the conclusion that **what you see on television is insane.** If you value your health you must not learn your meanings from television.

Our violent world is being blown out of proportion by television. It's all relative of course and what we have is bad enough, especially considering the increase in youthful crimes.

I object to the get-rich-quick con artists, the weight loss hucksters, the snake oil salesmen, the dozens of identical cars going around that identical curve, the multi-hundred dollar symposia, the psychics, the angry-matte-black instant ab machines, and all the $7 packs of inspirational tapes and pamphlets and books on sale in four installments of $59.95 each. I object to 30 minute infomercials, without even a pretense of programming, and I object to a government which has forgotten that the airwaves are a public resource ultimately owned by you and me, the free citizens of a free country. And whenever I want to cut a tin can in half I also miss my Ginsu knives.

Those strong jaws, tight buns, and empty "*sincere*" eyes tell me that life hasn't yet reached those people. It is also clear that these criticisms of commercials are trivial when contrasted with the moral emptiness of the programs themselves. They all aim for safe mediocrity, moral bankruptcy, and an inhuman blandness even in the midst of appalling violence. It is impossible to imagine personal growth of any kind in the face of the clanging emptiness of TV.

We cannot recover our sanity even in those moments away from television. How long has it been since you felt at peace on the earth? Even our evening jog is spent rehearsing the corporate needs of tomorrow's staff meeting. We build these mental towers automatically and little notice that what we have built is insecure, made of rapidly eroding speculation, empty of reality, and blinds us to everything around us.

Have you looked out the windows in the walls of your life lately? What season is it? The years go by and we don't see the new leaves of spring, nor the new birds hatching.

We haven't walked through drifts of autumn leaves since we were kids. We never notice the tree in our own front yard, even though we may have planted it ourselves years ago. What is happening to the earth? We have ceased to care. The subject is health, remember?

How long has it been since you embraced your fellow human beings? How long has it been since you seriously talked to your mate or children, with no agenda. You don't know the names of your neighbors, do you? All you know is their function in the dry as dust pecking order you are so concerned with through all the dry as dust days of your life. Look at one of those faces you see every day, really look at it! Look past the boredom and the pain. Isn't there something marvelous in that face?

If there is no love, no peace, no feeling of connection in all your thoughts, you are lost! The green of Spring touches only those who welcome it. The best thing you can do tonight is to turn to those around you with curiosity and love. That is where the mystery lies, not in that empty television. Open a bottle of champagne, and laugh!

# 11

## The Canticle of the Carbuncle

In the old days our family friend Doc Welby genially said, "*That's a carbuncle. It can cause blood poisoning. You can die from blood poisoning. Let's get it opened and drained so the pus comes out, and it gets a chance to heal. Put on some hot packs to bring the infection fighters in your blood to the spot. Try a fresh slice of onion on it. You'll be just fine.*"

In the somewhat newer, slightly more scientific days, Doc Daneeka told us, "*Let's cut it open so it can drain. Take some sulfa tablets to kill the germs. Put a hot pack on to get the blood, carrying the antibiotic, to the spot. Chances are the heat will keep it open to drain which is a good thing. You'll be just fine.*"

In even newer days, and slightly more scientific, our Doctor said, "*Let me give you a prescription for some penicillin tablets. You might speed things along if you took the time to hot pack it. It will likely open and drain which is a good thing. It will heal in several easy days. You'll be just fine.*"

Now we have arrived at recent medicine which is completely scientific. A physician you don't know says, "*That is a significant intrusion abscess within your skin. It might be walled off. It might*

*not be. It might enter the muscle tissue below the skin. It might not. It can shed some of the infecting agents such as bacteria. We're not sure which ones. Most common are streptococcus or staphylococcus. It could be anything else. Until we are able to culture the interior of that abscess we won't be able to know. It could have occurred because you scratched your skin. You might have been bitten by an insect. You might have pulled a hair when your skin was not its most sterile clean. It might be due to low body temperature due to leukemia, or perhaps AIDS. You might have diabetes. You might have any of a variety of syndromes which could open you to that kind of infection. It will be necessary to order many tests to determine your status. We should take an HIV test of course. We need a blood sugar test. We need a full blood count with a differential. We need some immune system chemical studies. We need to know your T-cell count. We had better check your body for other sites where your blood system might have deposited some of those bacteria to grow. If you have a heart valve problem this could lead to fatal sub acute endocarditis or valvulitis. We had better do a complete checkup. Let's include an electrocardiogram and an echo ultrasound of your heart valves. You should be just fine.*" Thus, for a carbuncle on your back, you are going to get a complete head to toe checkup. If there is even a minor suggestion of a heart murmur in Doc's stethoscope, or a benign mitral valve prolapse so common among so many, or if you should say "*Ouch*" if he presses too hard around your liver, or your kidney, or your spleen, then he's going to say, "*Oh Oh, Let's get a CT-scan of the liver and the spleen. We'll take a blood culture just to make sure you're not spreading bugs. I'll begin you on an antibiotic injectable and oral. I'd like to puncture the abscess with a fine needle and send some of the aspirate to the lab for culture and sensitivity, because the antibiotic we select, while likely to be fine, may be one the germ is immune to these days. So understand, please, that I have no way of knowing what you have, besides seeing that you have some sort of infection. There is a risk in sticking a needle into it that it may spread, but it's not likely since I'll start antibiotics. You could develop any kind of body infection and we'll need tests. Remember, because I have to guess at the infection and its type, I have to guess at the antibiotic. I can't be responsible if the antibiotic doesn't take and we have to change it. You aren't allergic to antibiotics are you? You could die from that too. I mean, it's your responsibility to tell me, in advance, of any reason I shouldn't be treating you. Now, sometimes these bugs can run away with themselves and spread so fast, no matter what you do, that you could die. You do want me to take an aspirate. don't you? There is a risk that the bug could enter your blood stream. And you do want an antibiotic right away, even though you could die from an allergic reaction to it? You understand that there may be many underlying causes for your abscess, and we may need to keep sending you for tests? Even cancer can cause immunity to drop. It could be the center of that lump, who knows? If you have a cancer you could die, you know that? I don't guarantee you'll get well because in medicine there are no guarantees, implied or otherwise. We never know. Physiology and fate are funny things. Oh yes, while we're waiting to find out the test results, and observe the changes under antibiotic usage, you might put on a hot pack four times a day. It's not good medicine but it might make you feel better. Remember that hot packs run the risk of burning yourself, and that could make for a serious scar or worse. If it's too cool, it won't help. We'll do our best to help you. Incidentally, there's a good attorney down the hall. He'll do just fine.*"

If you happen to take your carbuncle to an HMO or other mis-managed care organization today, it's possible that a stranger you hope is a doctor might take enough time to say, "*That's a carbuncle. It can cause blood poisoning. You can die from blood poisoning. The nurse will get it opened and drained so the pus comes out, and it gets a chance to heal. A hot pack might bring the infection down. Time's up. Gotta go. Bye.*"

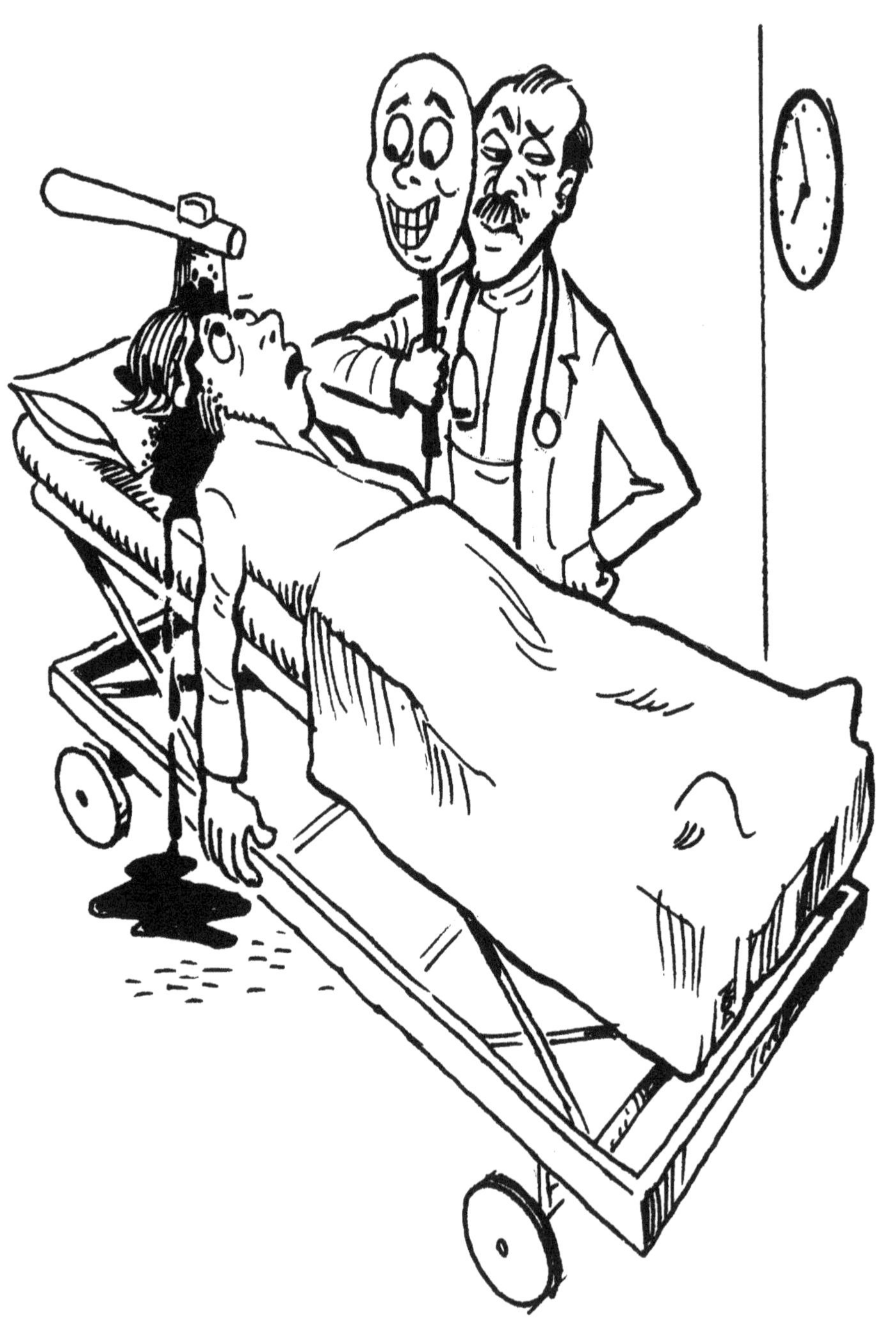

# 12

## The Politics of Mis-managed Care

Chances are you are less than 30 days away from bankruptcy. A week in the hospital and all hope of a comfortable retirement is gone. An operation is unthinkable. Any major disease and we are all broke.

Americans cannot afford medical care. Public Health Assistance mandates that we spend every cent that we have before we receive any. Congress doesn't have a clue. The assholes are stealing us blind! Congress and the HMO's hate Medicare although it's our only chance as we grow older. This is wrong. A sin is being committed. Pardon me if I sound a little old fashioned talking about sin this way. How can we avoid anger, and still respect ourselves and care about our world? Anger swallowed, anger denied, is our common lot today. What we need to do is to admit that all of us share my concern. We are all in this together.

Polls show we don't want HMO's. Tough noogies, Jack. Does your fire department have stockholders? As I write HMO's are being discussed, legislated, initiatives and referendums are being filed, mergers and takeovers are gathering steam, health care is volatile on the stock market, and the emperor has no clothes.

I hope you noted that it's not medicine anymore - it's "*healthcare*" - an amalgam of psychology, physiology, anthropology, epidemiology, education, management theory, and especially politics. What an opportunity for health economists to start thinking about "*quality of life*" for you and me. We can begin by conceiving of "*a universal outcome measure*" and begin to derive the "*quality adjusted life year*" (QALY) defined as the balance between life and risk measured as a number between 0 and 1. Health economists who are, of course, more economical of health than the rest of us, will declare this determination to be one that only health economists can make. You probably think I'm kidding dear friend. I'm not, you know.

I see talk show after talk show on TV, the last Town Hall in America, almost the last free speech off the NET - and see medical fear after medical fear expressed. Those ordinary people have the guts to get angry about all the lies, indifference, and neglect. What the corrupt old bulls see as a more than adequate national health care effort looks to the rest of us like a bandage covering a cancer. You are probably more afraid than I am.

The government wants "*the efficiencies of the marketplace*" in health care. The soul has gone out of "*our*" government and our influence is totally unimportant when compared with the cash laden influence from industry. Any questions?

Now it's time to discover the first of three Lesser Arcana dramatic productions to be found here and there in this book.

---

# MIS-MANAGED CARE

(theme music up to establish, and fade under voice-over:)

The Drama Department of Lesser Arcana Productions presents a heart tugging story of real life in America we call MIS-MANAGED CARE. All names have been totally changed to protect the innocent, if any.

As Scene 1 begins we see a patient we will call Woody (not his real name) sitting in a generic examination room, his rear end not quite covered by a hospital-colored gown. Doctor J. Voorhees (not his real name either) enters. Woody speaks:

WOODY: Gee I'm glad to see you doc. I was two hours out there in the reception room and 40 minutes in this closet...uh, I mean examination room. It gives a guy a lot of stress.

DOCTOR VOORHEES: Why? You have claustrophobia?

No. I need to catch a plane sometime and I can't spend all my life here.

Was that a wise crack?

No sir, just commenting on the truth. See, I sell tires, and if you had to stand and wait for me to put four new tires on your car, as long as I waited for you, I'd be having to sell shoes.

Can't you see I'm busy? We can't accommodate quick ins-and-outs when there are as many people as there are out there. And this is a slow day. What can I do for you?

Well doctor...mostly...see this is my sixth visit in three months. I'm getting more and more tired, and there's no reason for it, and each time I tell it to one of you docs, you tell me I'm probably working too hard. Now my wife is concerned. Says I'm even too tired to stay awake long enough to watch a game at night, you know, on TV?

So what's wrong with going to sleep?

Well...yes...but I don't feel good.

How am I supposed to know what "I don't feel good" means? Anything hurt?

No.

Anything ache, burn, feel upset? I mean gimme a clue and a break. "I don't feel good" is what little old ladies from Pasadena say.

Look doc, I'm 48 years old, not old enough to feel tired every day. I work out but don't even feel up to that any more. My wife says I'm depressed, you know, no sex and stuff. I could sleep all day.

Well, sounds like we have the diagnosis. Depression is common. I'll give you a prescription for Prozac and you'll be up and running in no time.

Doctor...If I'm truly depressed will you please refer me to a psychiatrist? I mean I want a real diagnosis, not just a pill.

Look, uh...,(refers to his clip board) Woody, We use consultants and specialists only where real trouble lies, and you haven't got it. Your last physical and lab were normal. Depression is as common as sore throat. Now tell me you want a specialist for a sore throat. Take the anti depression pill and start living your life. (starts writing out prescription)

Doctor...by the way you never mentioned your name?

(mumbling as he writes) Doctor Voorhees.

Doctor Hees, I'm telling you, I need a diagnosis. I'm depressed because I know I'm sick, not the other way around.

Hypochondriacs tell me that every day. (hands Woody a written prescription) Take this and see me in 4 months. (music under and up)

(voice over) And so Scene 1 of MIS-MANAGED CARE ends with action taken and Woody unsatisfied. When we return to scene 2 of Managed Care, after these words from our author, we will discover that all is not well with Doctor Voorhees. (music to end)

---

When Congress talks health, never being quite sure what they mean, being lawyers one and almost all, they toss around words like "*equal access for everyone*."

There's nothing wrong with the idea of equal access as I understand it, but the Congressional lawyers seem to forget the word "*everyone*," and in addition to efficient non-rationed non conditional illness care, it should also include access to a safe jog in the park, access to milk and clean vegetables, education, and awareness of the need for personal development for everyone.

Let's do some of that before our government commits to some half wit scheme without vision which actually reduces available health care quality in the name of spreading what's left over their version of "*equal access.*"

Prevention is a grand idea whose time has come but prevention cannot help all the old, the needy sick, and the impaired. These are not some useless crowd of strangers - I'm talking about your parents, grandparents, and maybe you.

We are dealing with the most pernicious promulgation of social Darwinism in our history. Baldly stated: "*If you are poor, you are inferior; therefore you deserve to die!*"

---

## MIS-MANAGED CARE

And now, from the Drama Department of Lesser Arcana Productions, here is Scene 2 of MIS-MANAGED CARE. You'll recall that Woody complained of constant tiredness and Doctor Voorhees had given him a prescription for Prozac and told him to come back in 4 months. We now go to the 25th floor corner office of Dr. Voorhees' boss. The HMO Administrator is speaking:

ADMINISTRATOR: Doctor Voorhees, I'm sorry to have to see you for the second time. Once more and we'll have to reevaluate our relationship with you.

DOCTOR VOORHEES: I'm sure that. . .

ADMINISTRATOR: You see, your specialist referral rate is too high. On the computed curve you refer six out of every 100 patients to some specialty. Now come on, doc! You have to have more confidence in yourself. The target is one in 100. At the target figure you will save five patients from consultations, which is so much money saved. So, to balance you out, no specialty referrals from you at all for the next three pay periods. It will allow you to catch up nicely.

VOORHEES: There's a good explana. . .

ADMINISTRATOR: And speaking of dollars and performance, I'll bet you didn't know that you ordered $3,200 more lab work this month than last. Just shows how medicine can get away from you if you don't pay attention, eh doc? That's $2,200 more lab per month than the average internist here averaged. During the next quarter you'll have to get under $2,500 or the computer will spit you out.

VOORHEES: Well, there's been an especi...

ADMINISTRATOR: I know you're busy but there's one more thing before you go. Your hospitalization days. Your patients have been in hospital 1.662 days longer than average. Too many hours here in hospital means too many wasted bucks. Hey doc, this isn't the old days when you just let it all hang out. I mean, if you don't pay closer attention to the bottom line of medicine, we'll be forced to chop your Christmas bonus. We don't want to get to the point where we have to chop you too, do we?

VOORHEES: Isn't there any flexi...

ADMINISTRATOR: I'm so happy we had this little chat doctor. Remember my door is always open. (music under and up)

(voice over) As Scene 2 of MIS-MANAGED CARE ends, a properly chastened Doctor Voorhees is prepared to apply himself anew to Woody's problems. Before we continue, let us pause for these words from our author. (music to end)

---

*"The Constitution of the Republic should make provision for medical freedom as well as religious freedom. To restrict the art of healing to one class of men and deny equal privilege to others will*

*constitute the Bastille of medical science,*" said Dr. Benjamin Rush, signer of the Declaration of Independence

We've gone a long way in America, from the profundities of Thomas Jefferson's generation, to the cue card manipulations of our latest president, to the man with the Smith & Wesson standing behind us at our ATM, ready to take our cash, our card, and all the health we have left.

Congress, with its alleged concern about health care, could easily begin by solving the tobacco issue. Then Congress could go on to the environment and its thousands of carcinogens and mutagens, and provide the job retraining, and the wherewithal, and the truthful commitment, to clean it all up, instead of trying to repeal or cripple even the pitiful efforts already funded in this direction.

Congress is afloat with half a life raft and no social direction, despite the 1986 Ottawa Charter of Health, or almost any issue of the New England Journal of Medicine, or the World Health Organization (WHO) guidelines. The information, in all its urgency, is easily available, and believe it or not, it is easy reading for lawyer/legislators. The problem is not understanding - the problem is corruption.

The United States is almost the only modern industrialized nation that does not have some form of national health insurance (South Africa does not). Polls have shown time and time again that Americans would prefer some sort of national health-insurance system, and time and time again it has been shot down with charges of "*socialized medicine.*" Universal medical care just isn't capitalism, and it grates on the stock market's nerves. This is America where insurance companies, and the clowns in Washington, tell you that proper preventive health care is too expensive, because everyone has to get their cut or it won't fly. That is the glaring truth of the health plans seriously considered by Congress. All of them make sure that no money interest or power center loses.

Cut down on your pap smears, your mammograms; as a soda beverage, a telephone, and a pair of pants spend 900,000 dollars for a 30 second commercial during a football game. "We seldom reflect that we already have "*socialized*" police forces, "*socialized*" elementary and secondary schools, and "*socialized*" fire fighters. You can't buy stock in any of them, and none of them are listed on the stock exchanges. The real question would appear to be whether medicine, too, should be a social service, or whether it should remain primarily a commercial profit-making business."[1]

You are probably totally confused by the media blitz from the HMO's - the We love you's and the We care for you's and the unmitigated unethical propaganda, most of it total non-sequitur - while you shiver in your boots over losing the little insurance you already have. Long term care pauperizes everyone, without exception, except the rich. We're all caught up in an epidemic spread of stupefaction and its associated illiteracy. Political, social, industrial, and personal incompetence is as virulent and as life threatening as that gang member's Uzi.

One of the first concepts those lawyers busy making laws were told in school is that laws without morals are in vain. By my senior year in law school this was considered sophomoric. A society of more laws than people is a tyranny.

Despite what television tells us, those damaged people in our multiplying prisons are not stupid. Like any human being, no matter how dehumanized, they probably retain a far-off golden memory of what might have been, a ghost of hope, peace, brotherhood, and their first plans of childhood. The longer we tolerate conditions that turn our brothers into animals, the sooner they will learn violent war in the streets. It is never the fundamentalists, the middle class, or the intellectuals, who first notice tyranny!

We look for reassurance, and who better to give it to us than our politicians, to whom we willingly hand over our minds? Who better than politicians to promise a better world to come? Who better than our army of marvelous bureaucrats to promise us our glorious destiny? Where better to put our trust?

There is no politician in the entire country with enough guts to remind anyone that 30 percent of America's medical expenditures are for emergency rooms, which are always cut first when hospital cost cutting time arrives.

The rapidly growing population of uninsured residents in L.A. County is now larger than that of any other industrialized **nation** except South Africa. The L.A. County Board of Supervisors now threatens to close the County Medical Center, adequate 60 years ago when it was built. They are talking of building a new hospital with

40 percent *fewer* beds! The spokesperson for the supervisors said this was "*a visionary nod to a future of improved technology and managed care that would continue to make hospital stays rarer and shorter.*" No doubt.

When government talks health I think of the old Roman saying: *Cui Bono*, which means Where is the good?, i.e. Who gets the profit? Which way is the bribery going? Who gets the cut? No matter what they say, my health is far down on their list.

The emergency room staff is exhausted, the police are exhausted, the firemen are exhausted, our schools are exhausted, and we are exhausted. The politicians are smiling. Who will make it perfectly clear that the barbarians have taken over?

---

## MIS-MANAGED CARE

And now, from the Drama Department of Lesser Arcana Productions, here is Scene 3 of MIS-MANAGED CARE. You'll recall that the HMO administrator had gently admonished Dr. Voorhees for unprofessional conduct. As Scene 3 begins Dr. Voorhees is seeing Woody once again:

DR. VOORHEES: Back in only two weeks instead of four months are we...uh, (refers to clip board) Woody?

WOODY: Yes, me.

Why are you on my back?

I'm on this table, doctor.

We're both depressed are we?

No, I'm sick! I'm tired, and I pissed blood yesterday!

(interested) When and how?

Just at the end of the stream.

Only a little?

Yes, but it scared me to death!

Well, you've probably got prostate swelling. Still no sex?

No sex. No interest.

Depressed, eh? OK, drop your pants and let me check your prostate.

(Woody bends over. In goes Voorhees' gloved finger.) Nothing there. Just a little boggy prostate from no sex. Do it or jack it, and the gland'll go down.

Doc, blood in my urine scares me.

Do as I say. Nothing to be concerned about. Have the nurse set up an appointment in two months. (music under and up)

(voice over) As Scene 3 of MIS-MANAGED CARE ends, we're beginning to be a little worried about Woody aren't we? Is he going to be all right? Will Dr. Voorhees get chopped? Only five more scenes to go, but before we go ahead here are a few words from our author. (music to end)

---

And on that note I begin my discussion of Health Mis-Managed Care Organizations (HMOs). What many HMOs offer in their glossy brochures are ways to get something for nothing. What they promise may be nothing like what some of them deliver. "*Tanstaafl!*" was the acronym Robert Heinlein used (There Ain't No Such Thing As A Free Lunch!).

A major study, soon buried, showed that most of you were not willing to accept an HMO. It is easy to forget that long before the

HMO controversies erupted, people were already far from happy at the spiraling costs of private medical care.

When HMOs first began expansion, you probably had in mind something like the credibly responsible non-profit Kaiser plan, still America's largest medical plan and still non-profit. What you got instead was the "*fast-food*" cheapo HMO industry where profit, not care, is paramount.

Over 70 percent of Californians are members of managed care groups. These figures will soon be matched in your state. A survey has found that 42 percent of Californians had a problem with their health plan in the last year, ranging from denial or delays in getting medical treatment, to inappropriate care, or difficulty in getting referrals to specialists. Twenty-one percent said the problem led to a worsening of their medical condition. It is difficult, and often impossible for financial reasons, for individuals, especially those retired and on Medicare, to leave their HMO. This hardly suggests that we are satisfied, as some have claimed.

It is clear that people want the right to freely choose their own *affordable* doctor who is responsible to them directly and has time to talk to them, not a conflicted doctor who's primary task is to make a profit for a security exchange listed corporation. A recent newspaper editorial said, "*The benefits of customer loyalty and improved long-term health care outcomes more than compensate for slightly higher costs for physician's time.*"

Increasing numbers of doctors (now five percent of the nation's 700,000 or so doctors) are joining unions. The president of the Union of American Physicians and Dentists says, "*What we want is the same as what everyone wants, we're working stiffs, too*". Solidarity Forever, eh doc?

---

## MIS-MANAGED CARE

And now, from the Drama Department of Lesser Arcana Productions, here is Scene 4 of MIS-MANAGED CARE. You'll recall that Woody had begun pissing blood, and Dr. Voorhees had been a little less than glad to see him. As the scene begins five weeks have gone by:

WOODY: Hi, doc.

DR. VOORHEES: Oh, no. Not you! Has it been two months already?

I'm bleeding. For two days now my urine has been red start to finish. I tried to stay away. I even masturbated. Bleeding! Still bleeding.

Well, I guess...Gee...You think it'll quit by tomorrow?

How would I know? You're the doctor. What is it that's bleeding? It sure ain't my gums!

OK. OK. Tell you what. Drink a lot of water. Could be you're passing a stone. Nothing hurts?

No.

OK. drink a lot of water, and come on back in two days...No, I leave on a three week vacation before then, first in a year. Come back in three days and Doctor F. Kruger will see you. (music under and up)

(voice over) Concern seems to be widening in Scene 4 of MIS-MANAGED CARE as Dr. Voorhees leaves our drama for a well deserved vacation. To reassure you, we'll let you in on a secret: Dr. Voorhees does not get chopped. Now here are more words from our author once again. (music to end)

---

Physicians "*may well end up, like tobacco company executives, representing their sins, finding their contracts forbid confessing them.*" The chief of a university hospital has reportedly admonished the faculty: "*Doctors who attract sick patients; for example, experienced surgeons, minority group physicians, medical school faculty members, and those who care for the poor, risk being ostracized from plans and even from physician groups, as the gulf between clinical excellence vs. professional success and profit & loss widens.*"[2]

We are hearing, as I predicted on the air years ago, chocolate coated words which mask the disenfranchisement of the elders, the young, or even anyone who has an expensive or preterminal disease.

Many private physicians regret the income reduction involved in treating Medicare patients, resulting in a massive shift of Medicare patients (old people) to HMOs, who quickly try to get rid of them in their turn. Shareholders want to participate in profits, not loss.

Managed care, "*is a blatant rationing scheme, intended to make doctors do society's dirty work. Why else is congress so eager to herd the elderly into HMOs? Ultimately, health care must become a regulated public utility.*"[3]

Independent doctors are trying to get HMOs to disclose exactly what payment method they use to pay doctors. They may not succeed.

Capitation is defined as a counting or assessing of each person (doctor), in this case an assessment for each non-recommended procedure, in other words each referral decreases the doctor's income. Many HMOs routinely keep 20 percent of their doctor's fees to be paid to him at the end of the year. Doctors who provide "too much care", i.e. too many tests, or process too many consultation requests, are penalized. The HMO may keep the 20 percent.

The average time doctors at some HMOs spend with their patients is 5.1 to 7.1 minutes. If you think this is happening to you be sure you, and your doctor, build a solid paper trail. Point out to management that procedures need to be done, not at the expense of the doctor, but for the benefit of the patient. The argument that capitation leads to dangerous undertreatment will be heard increasingly in courtrooms across the country.

It reminds me of the old stories of primitive tribes on the march, who kindly allowed their women to squat by the side of the trail to give birth, provided they caught up afterward.

Certain surgeries are denied, or dangerously delayed by some HMOs. Watch out if you need bypass surgery because of worsening angina. You may be delayed until you actually have a heart attack, and even then they may or may not do the indicated surgery.

Sometimes that terrible chest pain is only indigestion, or a panic attack. Sometimes it's a ripping aorta. Which it is can only be known in the emergency room. If it wasn't your aorta, your HMO may decide that you pay the bill. You, and not your doctor, must decide! Do you sense my carefully concealed fury as I dryly recount these atrocities, dear reader?

The health economy is being looted by "*HMO middlemen, parasites who skim off 20 to 30 percent, and add no value to the end product, create no real savings, and are awash with negative and/or perverse incentives...The insurance industry has become little more than brokers who dump their actuarial risks onto under-capitalized networks who pass it on to physicians and hospitals after skimming off huge profits.*"[4]

In 1994 and 1995 five Los Angeles HMO's refused to pay sales taxes they said were too high. The same five HMO's recently threatened to move out of town if a new request for lower tax rates was not met.

---

## MIS-MANAGED CARE

And now, from the Drama Department of Lesser Arcana Productions, here is Scene 5 of MIS-MANAGED CARE. You'll recall that Woody had begun pissing blood continuously and his doctor had suggested that he drink a lot of water. It is 3 days later and Woody is seeing Dr. F. Kruger for the first time. Dr. Kruger (not his real name) speaks:

DOCTOR KRUGER: So what brings you in?

WOODY: I'm bleeding in my urine.

How long?

All the time.

No, I mean how many days?

It's been over a week, and all the time!

Well I guess that qualifies you for a referral to a urologist.

Today?

You've got to be kidding. These guys are backed up with patients waiting. Probably about three weeks.

I'll bleed to death by then!

Look, here's what I'll do. I'll try to play a little politics. Today is Tuesday. I'll see if I can get you in by Friday.

Not now?

Sure, if you're carried in on a stretcher.

I'll take Friday. (He gets a Friday appointment, music under and up)

(voice over) As Scene 5 of MIS-MANAGED CARE ends it looks like Woody's bleeding problem is coming to a head thanks to a little rule stretching by Dr. Kruger who came into our drama just in time, and now leaves, never to be heard from again. The curtain will rise on Scene 6 after these carefully crafted words from your author. (music up to end)

---

I have heard it said that the complete annual physical is an idea whose time has gone. HMO's say that physicians are "*needlessly*" basing their preventive efforts on doing extensive physical examinations. How comforting those words must be for a profit oriented HMO.

The new wisdom is that all a physician should do is check your height, weight, and blood pressure yearly with a breast exam for women from 40 to 64, give you a visual acuity and hearing test, check on cholesterol only once a year, and spend a certain number of seconds asking if you smoke or exercise. Your loving family doctor is castrated (or hysterectomized).

We are being told not to spend any time and money on the patient! You can always say that a physical was unnecessary if it doesn't show something wrong, but what happens if you didn't do the physical and something wrong remains undiscovered? Necessary physicals are sometimes discovered posthumously. It can do a lot of damage to individual ~~customers~~, excuse me, patients, when you take away their physical exams. You don't treat an automobile that way.

The bean counters in Washington have recommended that we close a substantial percentage of the nation's medical schools, or limit the number of foreign graduates of American medical schools who can become residents of the U.S. The federal government has agreed to pay hospitals around the country hundreds of millions of dollars not to train doctors. The initiative, embedded in a federal budget agreement, extends to all 1025 of the nation's teaching hospitals an offer similar to one in place in New York state. All of this discussion is driven by the assumption that price, virtually exclusively, drives hospital competition. Some have asked, "*What about broader societal contributions, such as education and research, and what about quality of care?*" Measuring quality is not easy in the accounting department.

Teaching hospitals could not function without low paid medical residents. Cutting back and closing medical training institutions, while there exists an acute need for health care by so many Americans, remains difficult to swallow. While the ratio of physicians to population has gone up in the last 25 years, the number of medically under-served areas remains about the same. Congress has curtailed Medicare's commitment to subsidize the training of new doctors although some of the deleted funds are now reclaimed by teaching hospitals.

It has also been recommended that we significantly decrease the number of specialists. It goes along with political recommendations to diminish research funding while we are on the razor's edge of making major patentable breakthroughs in cancer and immune disease problems. Thanks to the politicians we are rejecting the exciting potential future of medicine in favor of election year tax reductions.

Any doctor today expects to hire a full time bookkeeper and government nursemaid in order to prove day by day, and soon minute by minute, that he or she is not a criminal. An innocent error can lead to a jail term. It's becoming a continuous kangaroo court trial, with no witnesses and often no legal representation allowed, and only one winner. Some patients may be allocated to physician's assistants, even nurses, and you're not sure who's taking care of you. I hear more and more horror stories of people who have escaped their mis-managed care organization just in time.

What all the "*indicators*" measure is control. The virtual vehicles traveling the infobahn include virtual tanks and virtual guns. We will all be having virtual netmares very soon. Yes, ladies and gentlemen, it **is** that bad!

Government repression is not only, or always, a gross assertion of control. More subtly, it may take the form of a demand for information, and the assumption of benign powers not proper or appropriate for government.

Medicine is presumed to be something every doctor worth his salt knows that it is not, a science! The law does not allow for human error, time spent getting to know your patients, or differences among people, in other words, the art of medicine.

The doctor will soon be running his own shoe store. The woman who asked for work washing windows, will soon be overworked making inexpensive medical decisions. The CEO is unavailable, he's sailing his yacht down the coast to Puerto Vallarta, past the Mexican urine testing labs. How much of your life are you willing to bet that this kind of story has no basis in fact? The top executives of America's major HMO's received more than six million dollars *each* in total compensation in 1996. I could find no more recent figures, but I doubt if compensations have gone down, The members of one major HMO paid an equivalent of 40 dollars each to the major executives of their organization. Compensation expert Graef Crystal said, "*When people see doctors' pay being reduced and nurses being thrown out on the street, as you wade through this sea of misery, you suddenly find yourself knee-deep in the plush-carpeted office of an HMO executive who's making millions.*"

We don't have much time left to turn the situation around. If we don't do so, our quest for health will become nearly impossible. Oceans of statistics don't help us to become healthier.

I am not advocating that our government cease protecting the public interest, defined very broadly. We will always need to be protected from the tobacco salesmen of the world. There are crooked and venal doctors here and there. What I am advocating is a careful differentiation between protection on the one hand, and interference with the private activities, and freedom of transaction, of consenting adults on the other.

You have seen some of the many editorials about mis-managed care, showing up in most of the nation's newspapers. Your state may have a lobbying group (or two) with a name like "*Citizens for the Right to Know*," or "*The Center For Health Care Rights*." There is a "*California Managed Care Improvement Task Force*" and your state probably has something like it. There are calls for state regulatory agencies devoted to managed care. A growing number of state legislatures are giving doctors and patients at least minimal rights to due process. Health plans that dump what they consider to be "*expensive*" doctors are increasingly being forced to justify their actions and affected doctors are even being given a fair hearing. There is some awareness of action needed to preserve rights of privacy in traditional doctor/patient consultations.

The American Association of Health Plans, an industry lobbying group, suggests that one way the mis-managed care industry might be able to kill or weaken reform efforts is by arguing that regulation will raise medical costs and taxes. Some of the same insurance and employer groups that used a similar strategy to help defeat Clinton's flawed health care reform plan in 1994 are campaigning to block attempts in Congress to set federal quality standards for health plans.

A group of three health maintenance organizations and two consumer groups, in an effort to stave off Congressional regulation proposed a "*Patient's Bill of Rights*" for the presidential commission studying the matter which then reissued the proposal under its own name. Meanwhile the health plans are keeping one step ahead of us with new ways to save money by increasing efficiency.

There is a major national controversy about HMO's under way. Congress is heavily involved. Legislation or public opinion may ameliorate the worst abuses but no matter what happens, we now know that the machine has no heart. Go back and re-read what I have said. Can you really say that my tone of high outrage is not justified? You and I are going to have to be terribly alert from now on.

---

## MIS-MANAGED CARE

And now, from the Drama Department of Lesser Arcana Productions, here is Scene 6 of MIS-MANAGED CARE. You'll recall that it took a late intervention from Doctor F. Kruger to get Woody a rare appointment with a specialist. As our drama continues, urologist Dr. M. Myers (not his real name) is just about to leave for the day. He is speaking to the nurse:

DOCTOR MYERS: Damn if it isn't late. I quit at 5:00.

NURSE: Just one more. You have 10 minutes to go.

MYERS: Just one? (turns and sees Woody sitting three feet from him)

WOODY: Hi.

MYERS: Yes?

I'm bleeding.

From?

My penis.

Hard sex?

No. All the time, with urine.

How long?

Seems like weeks now.

Well, guess you need a cysto.

Cysto?

That's looking in the bladder through the penis with a tube, look around, find bleeding.

God, that's awful. Up the penis?

You want help or not?

When do we do it?

OK, let's see. First Uro schedule I can get you is day after tomorrow. Be at the outpatient clinic at 5:00 AM. Nurse'll give you directions. We'll need to anesthetize it...

My penis?

Yes, your penis, and after the cysto you can go home in an hour. Probably better to have the wife drive the car home. (music under and up)

voice over) Maybe woody is beginning to understand that important matters are afoot, as it were. We'll be discovering what it all means in Scene 7, of MIS-MANAGED CARE coming up next, after these words from our author. (music up to end)

---

A better approach to public health care might be to give the citizen the right of choice of doctor and hospital with no right of refusal for bad risks. There are private group insurance plans. There must be a way to get premiums down by insuring the entire population of the United States, not just small groups. Canada has an interesting solution never seriously considered by most of the lawyers in Congress who tell us that Canadians don't like it. So does Hawaii. The lawyers are lying.

Physicians are on a collision course with professional liability claims. The severity of claims is increasing. Plaintiffs are beginning to win more often, and the significance of having a claim is rising. Part of the problem is that the expectation of the patient is at an all time high.

While physicians may have been to blame in the beginning, it is now the marketing departments of mis-managed care organizations which are getting the patients to believe the HMO doctors are gods in white, in order to increase profits. Most HMOs are portraying doctors as having all the time in the world to spend with patients. HMO enrollees mistakenly believe they are entitled to comprehensive high quality care with the very latest technology, promptly, and with magic attached. As these things don't materialize the patient then feels quite justified in filing a law suit for any potential bad outcome, small or large.

Plaintiffs lawyers are also spending more and more money on advertising, which will make many more patients think about filing claims. The consequence of having even a dismissed mal-practice claim intensifies with mis-managed care's growth.

Mis-managed care also severs the close bond between a physician and a patient and this incites patients to sue even more often. Some studies have shown that 80 percent of all malpractice suits involve a communication problem. Other studies have shown that physicians with a high frequency of mal-practice claims are those who limit office visits to less than 10 minutes. A patient feels rushed, rarely advised, tests are rarely explained, but it suits the mis-managed care format quite well.

It is expected that there will soon be another 286,000 events which could easily be brought to court against physicians in mal-practice claims. Another reason litigation will increase is that there is now money in deeper pockets than ever before. The market value of mis-managed care companies is in the billions. More and more cases will be filed for failure to diagnose, or inadequate treatment, rather than excessive treatment. Imagine what the cost of this is going to be.

Some lawyer is going to say to a physician, "*Hey, maybe it's time you filed a countersuit against the mis-managed care organization for being brought to court under these circumstances. Being forced by cost containment to produce poor patient care by the insurance company you work for should really be their fault.*"

The advanced degree in business administration for doctors being offered at the Irvine campus of the University of California is only one of dozens of similar courses being offered or soon to be offered at schools around the country, such as the MD/MBA programs at Tufts University, and Texas Tech. at Lubbock. These programs were begun to capitalize on physician's need for business smarts "*in a marketplace dominated by managed-care health systems.*" A member of the Commission on the Future of Medical Education at U.C. said, "*We are seeing the death of a cottage industry and the birth of the industrialization of medicine*". Another member of the commission, in noting that some doctors would resist these changes said, "*They fear we will lose many of the benefits that traditional medicine has brought us.*" To clear the air, note that the Oath of Hippocrates is printed in its entirety in Chapter fifteen.

Everybody is soon going to be suing everybody. It is impossible to practice good medicine in this environment. Physicians agreeing to a "*Hold Harmless*" clause, that most mis-managed care organizations are attempting to incorporate into their contracts, is making things very dangerous for physicians. They shift the risk of bad outcome directly onto the doctor, by obligating him to assume sole liability, by direction of the management of the HMO. Have you noticed that none of the above has anything to do with the underlying competence of the doctors involved? It's a legal, not medical, disaster in the making.

# MIS-MANAGED CARE

And now, from the Drama Department of Lesser Arcana Productions, here is Scene 7 of MIS-MANAGED CARE. As our drama unfolds it is 6:00 AM two days later, Woody is somewhere offstage in uro getting intimate with a cysto. We are with Woody's wife in the reception area. The coffee is powder. The cream is powder. The imitation sugar is powder. The magazines are a year old, except for the National Geographics which are 40 years old. The phone rings. The receptionist asks if Woody's wife is there. Woody's wife (not her real name) goes to the phone and speaks:

WOODY'S WIFE: Yes? Hello?

DOCTOR MYERS (on phone): Your husband has a malignant bladder tumor, and it's bleeding like a river. We'll have to take him up to surgery now. It's a tough decision but we may have to remove his bladder, and put in a special device. He'll dribble a lot but they learn how to control it after a while.

WIFE: Oh my God! At age 48! What are his chances?

MYERS: Look, who knows? Cancer is cancer, and he has been bleeding a lot, so he's a big risk. He can die now or later. I've got to go. He's bleeding and you don't want to just stand around when a guy is bleeding.

How will I know what is happening?

We'll call.

(three hours go by)

(phone rings as before) Yes - please?

I'm sorry to have to tell you this ma'am. Woody's cancer has spread. Wish we could have caught it earlier before it had a chance to grow into the bladder muscle. His is fast growing and it's way beyond just the bladder wall muscle. It has grown into the intestines and around the back wall. So...I guess you can take him home by day after tomorrow.

What can I do with him? Is there therapy?

Well, if we had gotten him early, maybe we could have hoped for a cure, but he waited so damn long to get help that he let it grow and it got away from him. (music under and up)

ANNOUNCER: (voice over music) I guess the moral of Scene 7 from MIS MANAGED CARE is be sure you get attention as soon as you notice something wrong and don't wait until it is too late to seek help. At least Woody has the consolation of a few days, or even weeks, to say his good-byes to his loved ones. There is one more scene left as we say goodbye to Woody. But that's after these words from our author. (music up and out)

---

All this reminds me of what we were taught about freedom in our schools. We believed it and internalized it, because it was beautiful. It's still part of our mental world and not to be disturbed.

Something nasty seems to be going on behind our backs. Jefferson's self evident truths are still truths to us, but not to our rulers.

Politician's ideas are settled by money, by a reelection donation, a subsidy in the pocket, management for an insurer, a lobby group. The resultant inevitably boils down to rationed health care.

Hospitals are closing. Is the latest cloud of smoke from the Ministry of Truth going to hide from us the reality of our own diminishing chances for quality care? We don't have enough money to keep the County hospital open but we are always able to pay for another press campaign extolling business opportunities. Is there a connection?

Our politicians who are not our representatives seem to think all doctors are greedy, selfish human beings, and should be done away with. Almost all politicians are lawyers (greedy, selfish human beings, who should be done away with). What will we have, after Congress is finished tinkering?

Moral law is embodied in great part in the physician's oath of Hippocrates (Chapter 15) as old and as outdated as it may seem to the world today. Moral law does not exist in concert with bureaucratic law, political law, or social law. Can the doctor serve two gods; the god that writes his check and the God within his patient?

All you want is the very best care you can get, so it may be important to note that most HMOs do not look kindly on outside medical opinion or surgical intervention even when more expert than their own. Coverage may cease in these cases and post operative care may be disallowed. Investigate "*point-of-service*" or "*open-ended HMOs.*" They're more expensive but more flexible about outside help.

Be sure you read the contract before you sign with an HMO, even if they make it difficult for you to do so. And where can we go to get unbiased information? Your state has a department that oversees HMOs. It could be called the Department of Insurance, the Department of Corporations, or the like, The National Committee for Quality Assurance recommended bringing all managed care plans up to the level of the best (1-888-275-7585). They won't tell you everything you want to know but they can help. They cover around 200 HMOs.[5] The National Association of Health Plans, representing 1,000 managed care groups, has a list of questions to ask before you pick an HMO. It might help to get a copy.

The unpleasant surprises are usually subtly coded somewhere in the small print, and can be found with close attention. Check your physician's credentials. Read books, talk to other doctors. Be sure your hospital has a good reputation. Some institutions have several times the survival rate for your operation than others do, and that information is sometimes available to the public with a little prying. Try your state government. At all points we must look for warning signs, signaled as much by what we are not told, as by what we are.

As a result of an agreement between the Federal Trade Commission and the nation's largest repository of medical information, the Medical Information Bureau (MIB), which compiles data for insurers, any insurance company must tell you if you have been denied insurance coverage, or charged a higher rate, because of an unfavorable MIB report. You can also get one free copy of your MIB report, usually costing eight dollars (at the time of this writing). The MIB estimates that more than half a million erroneous reports exist in its databases.

---

## MIS-MANAGED CARE

And now, from the Drama Department of Lesser Arcana Productions, here is the eighth and final scene of MIS-MANAGED CARE. We've reached the end. In Scene 7 Woody was given his death sentence. The bigger picture is revealed in this last scene, which takes place in the funeral chapel and at a phone in the anteroom. The organ is tastefully playing Nearer My God To Thee in the background as the generic Minister (not his real name) speaks:

MINISTER: God giveth, and God taketh away. It is written in the books of Heaven that the good patient Woody has gone to his deserved and eternal rest under Thy guidance and in Thy Holy... (fades down to continuing holy murmur in background as the HMOs stockbroker, Mario Millekun (nothing like his real name), speaks to his client on the phone in the foreground)

MR. M. MILLEKUN: "*. . . Some of the best growth stocks I can recommend are in the health care field. I'd recommend HMOs. Yes. They've been a little volatile lately but they're still a hell of a good investment. I just talked to an Administrator and they've got tight control over expenditures. It's a money machine. It packed away 65 million in profits last year, and it looks like it's going to be 111 million this year. They keep costs light. They have excellent handling of patients, with no waste, no unnecessaries. Good management. The CEO made 6 million dollars last year, and that's* *not counting bonuses. He really has that place humming with dough. A cash cow. They're in talks on mergers with several other HMOs. Dividends will grow like ivy. Buy it now and send your kids to college in style. I put all my own Keogh Plan and retirement money into HMO stocks, I know a sure fire investment when I see one. After all, I've been in the business since 1988. You're welcome ma'am.*"

From the Drama Department of Lesser Arcana Productions, the curtain falls on the 8th. and final scene of MIS-MANAGED CARE. I had fun naming our three doctors, F. Kruger, J. Voorhees, and M. Myers, after three of America's favorite motion picture characters. If you don't know what their initials stand for, ask anyone in their twenties or thirties who loved slasher movies. (music up to end)

THE END

---

If I am to embrace the things necessary for health, my discussion must wander into this grim and twisted darkness, and get involved in matters of power and national decline, corruption, and the priorities of a nation in pain. Sorry.

The tragedy is that I could not practice good medicine in the 90's, and I tried. This has nothing to do with Democrats and Republicans, and a great deal to do with the spiritual malaise affecting us all. Perhaps at other times in history it was possible to practice medicine divorced from the surrounding culture. It is no longer.

We are going down a road with a predictable end, and who is there to turn us aside?

Our government thinks we are children.

Robert Bork, when he was Solicitor General of the U.S Department of Justice, wrote these words, "*Beneficiaries of Medicare have the right to whatever the government sees fit to provide. Patients whose medical care is provided by public funds have no Constitutional rights.*"

Our rulers seem to assume that no one, here or elsewhere, values freedom or cares about the great dream of the (so young!) Founding

Fathers. They are wrong! Everyone, everywhere on earth, can understand freedom. There is a deep and rising discomfort beginning to come up to consciousness in America. **We are beginning to get angry** and we can't express our anger! It's called tension, and it's not good for our health.

*1 Ian Robertson, Sociology.*

*2 New England Journal of Medicine, 21 December 1995, p. 1706, Stephie Woolhandler, M.D., and David Himmelstein, M.D.*

*3 Dr. H. Rex Greene, Newsletter.*

*4 Dr. H. Rex Greene, Newsletter.*

*5 Modern Medicine Journal, headline story, August 1995, vol. 63.*

- *Dr. Ellen Taliaferro of Parkland Memorial Hospital in Dallas, Dr. Patricia Salber, Physicians for a Violence-free Society, publication: The Physician's Guide To Domestic Violence (214-590-8807).*

- *Robert Musil, Ph.D., exec. dir. Physicians For Social Responsibility, (202) 898-0150.*

# 13

# Your Immune System, Allergies, and Cancer

## Part 1: Your Immune System

The amount of cancer in America has been going down slowly since 1990 (I'll bet you didn't know that.) which may not help you and me. Still, we are no lightweights you know! We've got an immune system to defend us that has been developed and honed and made more powerful through billions of years. What counts is how we defend ourselves against the bad guys: bacteria, viruses, fungi, toxic chemicals, and inflammation.

We have a good rind, a good bark, on us, which doesn't help when things go in our holes. Even there, in the mouth, nose, eyes, sinuses, and down the digestive tract to the other end, we've got a lot of defenses. Past our crust our body waits, ready to pounce, to search and destroy. We have a miraculous armory and chemical factory ready to design and manufacture our troops at a moment's notice - over a trillion white blood cells, macrophages, lymphocytes, T-cells. Medicine will soon have other defenses against viruses, and most fungi, bacteria, toxins, and cancers as well. We are also learning new ways of sneaking past our skin, and into our bodies and brains with subtle and powerful medications.

The body's divine smoke, the antibodies, tangle the stranger and wrap it in a cloud of unknowing until the other protective cells, the lymphocytes, the macrophages, can do their work. The T-cells produce hundreds of antiviral, antitumor, anti-inflammatory chemicals, all mediated by chemicals sent throughout the body by various organs including the brain! Some of them are called interferons which (you guessed it) interfere, each with its own specific kind of virus. Our immune system even tries to protect us from the man made poisons everywhere in our world that were unknown when this miraculous system originated. It does not always succeed. Interferons are specifically manufactured by the thymus gland to destroy specific viruses at the moment of invasion. If everything is working correctly, when the interferon gun is fired the virus is destroyed. HIV and some other viruses keep the gun from firing.

Researchers have reported that contaminated water, food, and air are suppressing human immune systems worldwide, lowering our resistance to viruses, bacteria, and tumors we could otherwise have fought off. Autoimmune disorders are "*mysteriously*" (really?) on the increase.

Canada reports that Inuit (Eskimo) children, dependent upon the products of the polluted oceans for much of their food, have suffered a 20-fold increase in meningitis in the last few years as compared with other Canadian children. Their immune systems are so compromised that they sometimes fail to produce enough antibodies even to react to and activate the usual childhood vaccines.

A compromised immune system puts out the welcome mat. No one dies of AIDS. AIDS victims die of all sorts of other things we don't usually notice.

We don't dream of the number of times each day our immune system protects us from invasions. Plastic outgassing from clothing, carpets, etc., heated TV wires, your gas stove's pilot light, that light film of poison on the skin of your apple, smog, every microorganism known to man floating in the breeze, and a world increasingly full of metabolic poisons constantly attack us!

When I went to medical school, doctors cut out adenoids and tonsils and taught us the thymus was a useless appendage. Dentists pulled teeth as a matter of course, as an aid to whole body health. It was only recently that these allegedly useless structures have become recognized by medical doctors as very important parts of the immune system, appendix included!

Polychlorinated biphenyls (PCBs), DDT, and dioxin, are still carried in the tissues of every living thing on earth. The stories are horrifying. Our newspapers and television stations realize that we don't want to know, so they don't tell us.

You can see what our immune systems do for us by looking at what happens when it all stops. If it doesn't bother you too much, look at the body of a pigeon melting back into the earth, a day or two after its death. The soil of the earth is what we are, without our immune system.

## The Ballad of the Sweaty T-Shirts

One of those research studies that seem "grodie-to-the-max" may help explain why your immune system is as strong and complex as it is. At least I'd like to think that Claus Wedekind, a zoologist at Bern University in Switzerland and his colleagues, had something virtuous like that in mind when he had a group of 49 women, midway between their menstrual cycles, smelling sweaty men's T-shirts. Why not vice versa? Wedekind points to the increased odor in unshaved armpits. Ah, science!

To back up a bit, prior studies of female mice had shown that they tend to prefer the odor of their nestmates until puberty, at which time they go looking for the wild thing. Then when they get pregnant, they revert, and nest with relatives who can help nurse the young and protect them from strange smelling and murderous males. You can see the connection here already, can't you?

That's where the dank T-shirts come in. Humans, just like mice it turns out, can recognize differences in scent based on a group of immune system genes called Major Histocompatibility Complex (MHC), which are the most diverse of all human genes. No one has exactly the same ones. Women in the study tended to like the body odors that were most different from their own. The T-shirt odors they liked tended to remind them of former boyfriends.

In the interest of PC, maybe I'd better cut to the bottom line as quickly as possible here. Here's what it means to you and me. You've heard of hybrid vigor. Dissimilar MHCs, in one's parents, tend to broaden and strengthen one's own immune system! And it's quite possible that your mother and father may have been attracted to each other in the first place because, well, you know.

This is probably a good thing. Fertility is higher when genetics is dissimilar in our parents, miscarriages are lower, disease resistance is higher, and it turns out we can smell it all! No wonder there are taboos against incest. Deodorant and perfume manufacturers take note.

Did I mention the birth control pill yet? It raises estrogen levels in the body the way pregnancy does. Women in the study who were on the pill, preferred T-shirts with MHCs similar to their own. Like pregnant mice, they may prefer to be with ~~litter-mates~~, sorry, family members, with similar odors.

I won't ask what happens when sugarbuns and dear decide they should have children and she goes off the pill - and those wild genes down the street start calling. We like to think of ourselves as rational beings, very different from simple mice, so there's something a bit humbling in all this.

How can we possibly call medicine a science, in a world where the fact that your mother and father liked each other's smell when they were just slightly rank, may have as much to do with whether you catch a lot of colds, as the quality of your nutrition. Better not find someone to get engaged to until you've been off the pill for awhile. Think of the kids. Talk to me in 200 or 300 years about the science of medicine. In the meantime, as far as I'm concerned, it's an art.

**Part 2: Allergies**

Well that was fun, and it illustrated how complex and miraculous our bodies are, but it's time to move on to allergies. Allergies begin with the intake of a protein into our body. Many of the things that we're allergic to may be "*grody*" but they don't really hurt us otherwise, such as the pollens, the microskeletons of mites and the mite feces that make up dust, the hairs of animals.

The reason why conventional medicines don't always work is because an anti-allergy pill simply tries to suppress the system, which reacts ever more intensely by rebound and causes a great deal of toxic inflammation.

Some people, under acute emotional pressure get an outbreak of severe hives; nose, eye, skin, reactions; and there are people who can put their hands into ordinary kitchen detergent, or wear newly dry cleaned clothes, and exhibit the same allergic symptoms. A doctor treating hives has a thousand possible causes to consider.

A study exists in which plastic roses were brought into a room containing a group of people allergic to roses. Almost 90 percent of them reacted as if they were real roses, and became tearful, sneezing, stuffy nosed. They asked that the artificial "*roses*" be removed.

The research demonstrated that the attitude, the expectations, and the learned responses of a person has much to do with immune body behavior in addition to the actual proteins of the rose.

A similar thing happened with a broadly allergic woman patient. She had been to many doctors but the real truth was she hated her husband. After 11 or 12 years of marriage I finally, in discussion, discovered that. When she filed for divorce and separated, her allergies separated as well.

There is some journal literature that suggests hypnosis can completely prevent allergic reactions. This means that the hypnotist is teaching the immune system something!

The best answer is probably to combine all approaches. Reduce proteins of all kinds, clean up your surroundings, wash the cat, get psychotherapy of one kind or another, and take the prescribed injections. And beware of allergic emergencies which can be fatal.

Our interventions may disturb delicate balances. Before we take medicines to bring down fever we had better assume, in the absence of wisdom, that a fever might have a healing purpose. A fever may reach a band of curative discomfort just under our lethal level.

The same things can be said of eye strain, for instance. Temporarily elevated blood supplies to the affected region may be needed to carry poisons away and reconstruct damaged tissues. We may not be doing our eyes a favor by pharmacologically constricting this curative action in order to remove the redness. Permanently varicosed veins in the eyes are a possibility.

This gets pretty intimate. I don't suppose we are willing to give up cosmetics and dyes, but there are spectacularly harmful chemicals to be found in them. The skin is permeable to certain carrier chemicals. Entire commercial laboratories are devoted full time to discovering new products to apply to our exteriors. In any case do we really need 60 different products to clean, coat, pack, hide, scrape, bleach, oil, moisturize, brush, digest, dissolve, and color every square inch and orifice of our body?

There are many other subtle ways in which the body interacts with the world. Dancing with the moon, all women re-create the primal waters of the earth in preparation for conception and birth. We should carefully consider any intervention in these ancient rhythms. I'm not sure we really need all the douches, vaginal insertions, pills, and technical contraptions being used today. I'm not sure yeast infections would occur if we had not meddled with Selene to begin with. Too often we upset delicate and complex balances and then must deal with the results. Restraint is needed.

**Part 3: Cancer**

Pancreatic cancer has no cure. There is of course a treatment. It always results in failure, yet being mainstream, it is authoritative and not quackery. It is alleged to be good conservative therapy which recognizes it is dealing with a dying patient who can't be helped in the long run. It permits a patient to "*die in a traditional manner*", to die by the "*standards of the community*". It protects the patient from a quack - and the doctor from a lawsuit.

If you want to talk about quackery, how about the term "*bio-electric medicine!*" **Wowee! Zappo!** Orgone boxes, animal magnetism, and Frankenstein! Just the sound of it is quackery isn't it? Yet, it is now approved by the FDA to help heal broken bones in half the time it took before. So, I ask - is "*bio-electric medicine*" in conflict with the traditional orthopedic kit: 1.) the break, 2.) the cast, and 3.) the crutches; or would you say it might be "*complementary?*"

Is it quackery for desperate people to try innovation? Who cares whether it's quackery, if you're dying! What is rational in the face of certain death? That's what pancreatic cancer patients need to ask. It's what AIDS patients ask.

Today we stand somewhere between death and life and the needs of a medical science still struggling out of the muck of the ages. It is easy and comforting to say we are entering a medical golden age, but perhaps we should note where we stand now, at the beginning of this long climb. Everyone knows one or two lines of Thomas' great poem: "*Do not go gentle into that good night. Rage, rage, against the dying of the light!*" Everything becomes quackery until we have passed beyond it. Let us talk about our ignorance.

---

## THE EPIC OF ELOISE

The small and tasteful bronze plaque outside the huge impressive pile of distressed concrete and bronze tinted glass, over on the affluent side of town, says something like "The Academic, Mindbogglingly Well Known Institution of Higher Learning and World Renowned Experimentation" (the AMWKIHLWRE). You feel poorer just walking in the door.

ANNOUNCER: Here, from the Drama Department of Lesser Arcana productions, is THE EPIC OF ELOISE, one of the million stories from the AMWKIHLWRE which you can disbelieve at your peril. It was a dark and stormy night, and I was sitting with my feet on my desk, a bottle beside me (water). Then *she* undulated in. Eloise (not her real name) told me, "*Doc, I have had this pain for a few weeks in my lower abdomen. Then I began having bleeding. I went through menopause 3 years ago so this isn't likely. My husband says let's take your vagina into the ER and find out what's wrong. I thought that was a good idea. I got there at 7:30 PM,*" she said, "*and here's what happened.*" (Scene 1 of the Epic of Eloise:)

RECEPTIONIST: What's the matter?

I'm bleeding from my vagina.

So? Use a Kotex.

There must be an illness and I need to know what's going on.

You're one of the "worried well." That's what I tell most neurotic women who have one reason or another to show up here, especially at the height of the evening rush hour. Vaginal bleeding is no big deal, unless you're a man. Isn't that so?

Ma'am, I don't know. Since I had my last period three years ago, it's kind of scary to have one now, when I thought I was through.

So maybe you're pregnant.

Pregnant? I'm menopausal! My husband is vasectomized, and both of us are so busy being depressed and culture shocked we haven't fucked in eight months!

So, who've you been affairing with?

What an insulting comment.

OK. OK. Where's your insurance card? We can't see you without an insurance card or a deposit of 10,000 dollars for the first visit.

Eloise presents a registration certificate in the Republican Party and two insurance cards.

Two insurances, huh?

Yes.

You don't trust them, or you didn't pay the premiums of one of them?

They are both good.

Let's hope they cover enough. What's your name?

My God! It's on that license I just gave you.

Yes, but I just gave your ID to the clerk to get it photocopied and I'm facing the computer, so answer the question. Name? Address? Citizenship? Willingness to go to arbitration instead of malpractice court? If you say NO we can't see you.

Yes.

What's your problem?

I told you.

I'll bet you ate pork for dinner. You know, every time I eat pork I have a stomach ache. Barbecue it?

What? What did you say? Barbecue?

The pork. Did you barbecue it?

I ate sea bass.

Could be bad for you, especially if it swam in mercury filled water, or if they didn't refrigerate it soon enough. Why, you could have a case of indigestion.

And bleed from my vagina?

Oh, yes. You say you're not pregnant?

At my age? Lady I am going to bleed to death if you don't get me to a doc.

Don't get huffy with me! You ain't the only one here you know. See that room out there? There's 49 people ahead of you and if you want in there, you'll not raise your voice at me. What else bothers you?

Stomach ache, cold sweat. Come to think about it I might be losing weight these past three months.

That's great. I've gained 21 pounds. What's your secret?

Maybe cancer of the uterus.

Nah, I wouldn't choose that. Jenny Craig is safer. Please list your bank accounts here on this slip, savings and checking, your broker, and your mortgagor, and your car (owned, leased, and how much). Who will sign for you if you can't pay and your insurer won't?

Is this really necessary?

Yes, it's necessary before you can get into the ER care room. We take all necessary precautions. Now here's your number - 63.

I thought you said there were only 49 out there?

Well I just looked at the computer and there's been some come in by car, taxi, ambulance and one by helicopter in the last few minutes, and this isn't the only check-in desk, so now there are 63. Now please go between those two metal bars. We don't allow guns you know.

But if I walk much more I'll leave a path of blood. It's really coming now.

Look lady, either you cooperate with our rules or go somewhere else.

ANNOUNCER; End of Scene 1 of our little drama, brought to you by the Drama Department of Lesser Arcana Productions. You thought doctors didn't know about this sort of thing didn't you? It's just that we have problems enough of our own, getting good care to you, past all our own bean counters, without fighting your paper battles too. All of us are fighting a losing war for a little human dignity.

Lest you relax too much, I have to warn you that there's more to THE EPIC OF ELOISE. In Scenes 2, 3, 4, and 5 we've got to get

Eloise through the night. It all comes to a tired anticlimax around 7:30 AM the following morning. More after these words from our author.

---

Cancer runs along family lines under certain circumstances. No one is sure exactly what it is that is inherited however. We call it a predisposition, and we speculate about genetic defects, and occasionally identify a suspicious microorganism, or a gene, perhaps an "*oncogene*," which might be turned, by some triggering agent, into a cancer gene.

It takes the gene, the predisposition, plus something else in the environment, some "*X*" factor, one or many triggering agents. Doctors and researchers are now correlating triggers. They are everywhere, and include copy machines at work, solvents and laundry cleaners, tobacco, alcohol, auto exhausts, plastic outgassing, fat, protein; food additives including the nitrates and nitrites in pickles, pastrami, and luncheon meats, etc.; cosmetics, dyes, molds, certain preservatives, herbicides, pesticides, etc. Our immune systems are becoming increasingly overstressed by chemical and radiological attacks everywhere in our environment, usually minor in each case, but adding up unbearably. Notice how many of these triggering agents are man made.

Cancer of the colon, which might begin from a polyp growing in the colon, or breast cancer, seem to be genetically predisposed. We can nearly say with certainty today that if you haven't inherited the predisposing gene for colon cancer, you will not get colon cancer. Tests will soon be able to check a growing fetus for this predisposing gene. Some people will quickly add another reason for abortion to the list our grandchildren will inherit.

Evidence is mounting that aspirin and other nonsteroidal anti-inflammatory drugs may cut colorectal-cancer risk, no evidence that they will help reduce ovarian cancer risk. A newer study now seems to show that daily use of acetaminophen (but not ibuprofen) may cut risk of ovarian cancer as much as 60 percent.

Sunlight may cut colon and prostate cancer risks. **Lest you rush to complicated theological visions of massed ranks of naked elders mooning the rising sun, let me hasten to explain further.** (I can't believe I just wrote that sentence!) Researchers have announced that moderate exposure to sunlight anywhere on the body (!) may protect against the development of several types of cancer, even melanoma! This of course is heresy and should be carefully evaluated with your own doctor. I'm sure the operative word is "*moderate*".

Folic acid may also help control cancer and stop certain birth defects. Even though the U.S. government now mandates Folic acid supplementation in some foods, the amount will still be too low according to many Folic acid researchers. Check with your doctor as to the amounts you might need to take.

Men with prostate cancer have lower blood levels of the hormone form of vitamin D than age matched men without prostate cancer. Maybe we could also take a vitamin D supplement!

Men are happy to learn that there is minimal connection between an enlarged prostate and cancer of the prostate. Tests for prostate cancer are getting more sure. They don't involve biopsy (cutting samples) as often. Ask about the PSA test. Older men, especially those with a history of prostate cancer, and African-American men, should check regularly.

Women exposed to elevated female hormones (especially estrogen) have a higher risk of triggering the genetic predisposition to breast and other cancer. Birth control pills, and osteoporosis prevention drugs, are reasons for elevated hormone levels. Women who start contraceptive use by age 18 or before and continue for more than 10 years have a triple risk of developing breast cancer! Women can reduce their estrogen level by carefully monitoring the content of their doctor's prescriptions, reducing consumption of meat and animal fat, and upping vegetable intake.

Most gynecologists will tell you it's a bunch of baloney. Gynecologists say that adding the progestin pill will reduce breast cancer risk. There's a new study by researchers at Harvard, that says the risk of breast cancer in women who are taking progestin with estrogen is not reduced. Ask your doctor to keep up to date on this.

# THE EPIC OF ELOISE

ANNOUNCER: From the Drama Department of Lesser Arcana Productions, here is Scene 2 of THE EPIC OF ELOISE and her urgent vaginal bleeding. Eloise is reading material given her by a woman dressed in white (who is a real nurse, by the way).

Nurse: Yes?

Eloise: Yes what?

Yes, what are you doing here?

It's on all these papers.

Those papers don't mean anything.

Then why do they print them?

That's their problem. What's yours?

I'm vaginally bleeding.

Try a Kotex?

No. Listen, I'm menopausal. It's not normal bleeding. I hurt in my stomach, and it's not pork chops. I need help before I bleed to death.

Pork chops! Where do you lay persons get your ideas? So? You're not bleeding to death yet.

Can I see a doctor?

Don't rush me. What reason is there to see a doctor when I can do just as well. You're kind of pushy lady.

Help me before I die!

Get out of your clothes and put on this paper gown and lie down on that gurney.

Undress in front of everybody?

No. Pull the damn curtain lady, and tell your husband to go back and sit in the waiting room. It's busy enough here. The doctor will see you soon.

But it's midnight. When is soon?

Whenever they call your number.

My number is 63.

Well then probably by 3:00 AM. Try to snooze. It's a little busy here and noisy. It would have been better if you had an ear infection but nobody listens to me any more.

ANNOUNCER: So ends Scene 2 of THE EPIC OF ELOISE, brought to you by the Drama Department of Lesser Arcana Productions. There are three more layers of this confection yet to come, after these words from our author.

---

Even without an inherited genetic predisposition and all the poisons out there, the various X-ray and other ionizing radiation we have been exposed to may have knocked a DNA molecule askew here and there in our body.

I'm surprised to find that not many people my age have cancer in their feet. When I was a kid, many shoe stores had "*modern*" foot X ray machines, sometimes on the sidewalk outside, complete with a convenient eye level fluoroscope so you could see your bones. You stepped on them, like an old fashioned weight scale, to get your dose. The radium in them is still busily ticking away in land fills everywhere.

Dental X-ray films and fluorescent screens are much more efficient today. Even so we are always balancing advantages vs. harm when we have an X-ray. In addition to cancer, ionizing radiation can lead to diminished immune system efficiency.

In fact we will probably never be able to totally remove this cause of sickness because even stray cosmic rays going through our bodies seem to have some, as yet unmeasurable, and probably necessary (sub specie eternitatis), effect. In addition we are worrying now about industry's intensive efforts to thin the ozone layer, which can lead to an increase in malignant skin cancer for those exposed to undue amounts of sunlight.

There are a lot of sources and kinds of radiation we don't think about. Many smoke alarms work because they contain a source of ionizing radiation. Your television set is another source. We've all been alerted to radon gas in our homes. Ionizing radiation harms us primarily through the production of free radicals.

Each individual radiation source and chemical affront, we are assured, is totally harmless. They all add up. There is no "*safe*" dose beyond a certain irreducible minimum necessary for life to exist at all, despite what our betters say.

---

## THE EPIC OF ELOISE

ANNOUNCER: It's time to support the arts with Scene 3 of THE EPIC OF ELOISE and her urgent vaginal bleeding, brought to you by the Drama Department of Lesser Arcana Productions. We seem to be making progress. As this short transitional scene begins, we hear a real doctor (an intern) for the first time. He is speaking:

I'm Dr. Jones.

Eloise: Yes and I'm bleeding to death.

Let's not exaggerate now young lady. You look quite alive.

But not for long.

Tell me your name, age, date of birth, family history of bleeding to death. Do you smoke, eat sugar, drink booze, use crack, or pot? And when was your last flu shot?

Doctor . . .

I don't have much time. If you won't cooperate I can't see you. How many children?

Three. Doctor my thighs are sticking together from the blood.

We'll have the nurse clean you off later. Please answer my questions. Do you have any hobbies or redeeming social features? Oh, excuse me . . . It's 2:00 AM and I'm off duty. Dr. Smith will see you shortly.

ANNOUNCER: So Scene 3 of THE EPIC OF ELOISE and her urgent vaginal bleeding ends on a note of hope. We will return to Scene 4, from the Drama Department of Lesser Arcana Productions, after these few words from our author.

---

Recently, a defective gene was discovered which is the cause of a disease called "ataxia telangiectasia" (A-T), suffered by its carriers.

Not many people get A-T because the gene needed is only carried by one percent of the population, and it's recessive. You don't get it unless both your parents get a copy. That's not the problem. What if only one of your parents has the defective gene? You're not going to get A-T, but If you are a woman, your chance of getting breast cancer is suspected to be four or five times greater. The gene is also believed to be linked to a two or three-fold increase in your chance of getting melanoma, stomach or pancreatic cancer, and perhaps others as well. One percent of the population is well over two million people! No matter who you are, if there's someone in your family who's had cancer, you have a higher risk of getting the disease.

Other risks for breast cancer include being older than 60, beginning menstruation before age 12, having no children or giving birth to a first child after the age of 30, and a history of "lobular carcinoma in situ".

Sandy Kanicki, co-chair of an advisory panel to the National Surgical Adjuvant Breast and Bowel Project in Pittsburgh that recently conducted a new trial of the old drug tamoxifen says, "*The results are so profound that I'm speechless*". Does tamoxifen prevent breast cancer? "*The answer is an unequivocal yes,*" says Richard Klausner, director of the National Cancer Institute. Further study is underway.

As you should expect, tamoxifen has some pretty bad side effects, mostly in older women, chiefly a higher than average chance of developing uterine cancer and blood clots! In the past use of the drug has been limited to five years with effectiveness dropping off after that time. Breast cancer kills 43,500 American women each year. Should women who are at risk start taking tamoxifen while they are still healthy or would switching to a low fat diet do even more for them? Talk it over with your doctor.

Yet another gene is now being discussed. It's called BRCA2 and, like BRCA1, women having mutations in either have an 80 to 90 percent chance of getting breast cancer. The BRCA1 lawyers are eyeing the BRCA2 lawyers, so there may be something (expensive) in it.

Scientists at 87 medical facilities in the U.S. and several European countries are encouraged by the results of very early trials of an antibody treatment for breast cancer and possibly ovarian cancer. A few metastasized breast cancer patients have lost all trace of their disease! The treatment, sometimes in conjunction with chemotherapy, is aimed at the 25 to 30 percent of breast cancer sufferers who overproduce a protein that makes their tumors grow faster, produced by the "*HER-2/neu*" gene (I suppose there must be a "*HIM-2/old*" gene lurking somewhere). The antibody may be ready for use in a few years.

In another approach, UCLA researchers are going to be testing a new vaccine (!) against human "*glioblastoma*", an invariably fatal brain cancer. In early tests vaccinated rats were injected with 100,000 brain cancer cells, about 20 times the dose that routinely kills laboratory rats. The rats were not affected. Cancers of the brain, breast, lung, colon, and prostate all secrete a substance called "*transforming growth factor-beta*" (TGF-B) which suppresses the immune system and protects the cancer. The vaccine stops the tumor cells from making TGF-B. The research is in its very early stages.

The moral in these cases is clear: Do anything and everything to keep from getting your cancer for a few years until all this research leads to clinical practice.

There's a lot out there in our environment that may play around with our genes. Both men and women should steer clear of environmental triggers. Men exposed to elevated male hormones need to worry as well. Some effects take years to develop, or to make themselves obvious.

The culprit could be one of thousands of industrial "*endocrine disrupters*" (estrogen imitating chemicals). The evidence suggests that endocrine disrupters are the cause of falling human sperm counts around the world, female birds that act like males, male alligators with shrunken penises (there's something poignant about an alligator with a shrunken penis) and birth defects, and reproductive failures in everything from polar bears, to frogs, to Great Lakes fish. Perhaps I should also mention that farmers, exposed to agricultural chemicals, have lowered sperm counts as compared to non-farm workers.

You've probably heard about the Minnesota frogs with deformed or extra legs. It's probably a parasite infection but we don't really know. In a page one newspaper story about research in this being conducted by David Gardiner and Susan Bryant, biologists at UC, Irvine, it appears that offending chemicals may be hormone-like substances called retinoids. The story says that, "*Retinoids are found in humans, frogs and other vertebrates naturally, and are produced by lake plants and other natural organisms. They also can,*" and here the story is continued on page 24, "***come from pesticides.***" In excess, retinoids are known to cause deformities in human embryos. For example, pregnant women are told not to use retinoid-based skin creams."

Several studies in Europe in the last few months suggest that endocrine disrupters are causing a range of reproductive disorders that have become increasingly common in men worldwide, including testicular cancer, lowered sperm counts, undescended testicles, and urinary tract defects.

All of us are beginning to worry about endocrine disrupters. The problem is apparently not from the estrogen "*inhibiting*" chemicals in foods such as soy products, cauliflower, broccoli, and the like. These chemicals, rapidly degraded in the body, seem to confer protection against some forms of cancer, and have other protective functions. A plate of vegetables is fine.

The worry comes from the presence in the environment of long lived man made estrogen "*amplifying*" (not inhibiting) chemicals found in certain pesticides, drugs, fuels, and plastics, and industrial pollution in air and water. This is no surprise. We've been worried by these chemicals ever since World War II. There seems to be increasing information that breast cancer may be caused by these synthetic endocrine disrupting compounds. All other risk factors, including x-rays and genetic causes recently publicized, account for only about one third of all cases of breast cancer.

One of the most common sources of synthetic endocrine disrupting compounds is animal fat, corn oil and other polyunsaturated fats! Air and water pollution by industry is another major source. DDT, for instance, still persists in all environments and is still used, even today, in many developing nations which may export meat to us without our knowledge.

The long life of artificial estrogen mimicking pollutants is one of the major reasons why they are dangerous. They may enter the body only in small amounts but they are degraded so slowly that they may persist and accumulate for decades.

One Canadian researcher dissected beluga whales to see why their populations were declining. He found thyroid cysts, cancers, and tumors of all kinds everywhere in their bodies. One had bladder cancer like some of the workers at the aluminum plant on Quebec's Saguenyay River, a tributary where some of the whales spend a good deal of time.

The bodies of the whales contained high loads of industrial chemicals. One young whale had a concentration of PCB's 10 times higher than it would take to classify the animal as hazardous waste, under Canadian law. Is it necessary to dump these chemicals into our life support system? Does short-term private gain always outweigh long-term common good? And industry cries for less government regulation! There is evil here.

I suggest you buy and read "*Our Stolen Future*" by Theo Colborn, J. P. Myers, and Dianne Dumanowski. I also suggest you stop your daily ramble long enough to seriously consider your reaction to a world out of control, and lethal. **Isn't it time something was done?** How much longer can corporate propaganda persuade us to ignore our health and the health of the earth? Excuse me. I have to go into the attic for a while and scream!

---

## THE EPIC OF ELOISE

ANNOUNCER: As Scene 3 of THE EPIC OF ELOISE concluded we were led by Dr. Jones to expect the imminent entrance of Dr. Smith. As Scene 4 begins, brought to you by the Drama Department of Lesser Arcana Productions, Dr. Smith is speaking:

Hi there. I'm Dr. Smith. Why are you here?

Blood.

Blood?

Yeah. All of it coming out of my cunt.

Watch your language lady. Had a few tee many martoonis have we?

No. I'm just dying.

You said blood in your . . . uh, vaginal area?

I don't have a prick.

My. My. How long have you had this hostility problem?

Look man. If you don't get fucking ready to find out what and where I'm bleeding, and do something, either my husband or I will beat the living shit out of you! Can you understand that?

Threaten me once more madam and you get transferred to the County Jail. I don't need your abuse, you know.

ANNOUNCER: So, as Scene 4 concludes, we arrive at a crisis in THE EPIC OF ELOISE and her urgent vaginal bleeding. We invite you to look forward to Scene 5 and an effort, by the author, to find a way to save the situation for Eloise, although the Drama Department of Lesser Arcana Productions must remind you that nothing is certain in this best of all possible worlds. Now to a word from our author.

---

Infertility drugs seem to add to the problem. Women who take them for at least a year have a risk of ovarian cancer that is 2-1/2 times that of untreated infertile women, according to researchers. Cause is not proved but the correlation is suggestive.

Balance is all. If everything in your life is cancer skewed, you may die. If nothing in your life is cancer skewed, you will probably live. There is no science of cancer balances that will predict what happens in between. But notice that half of the criteria above are outside of our control, or if you are an optimist, half of them are within our control.

To keep it all in balance, note that about 15 percent of lung cancers appear in non-smokers. And about 85 percent of smokers never get lung cancer. Your genes determine how the body copes with what is done to it. Scientists believe there are scores of "*polymorphic*" genes that affect, either positively or negatively, our chances of getting the various insults that life can throw at our body.

It's quite clear that the first users of "*genetic profiles*" will be, not you, but insurance companies, mis-managed care organizations, and all the institutions of government control. If your printout shows too many "*cancer genes*" and "*polymorphic*" genes of the wrong sort, prepare for assigned risk, low care, high cost, and relegation to the low priority end of the mod med biz, and job hiring practices.

Welcome to *Ubermensch Triage International, AG.* (symbol UTI on the NYSE).

---

## THE EPIC OF ELOISE

ANNOUNCER: Television has just scratched the surface of the dramatic possibilities inherent in the health care field, as witness our continuing EPIC OF ELOISE and her urgent vaginal bleeding, brought to you by the Drama Department of Lesser Arcana Productions. Scene number 5 delivers us from tension, if not evil. The author has found a way to put the fault where it really lies. As the curtain rises, the Head Honcho of the Emergency Room, the Big Cheese, The Man, is approaching Eloise. It is 5:00 A.M:

Good morning. We've been bleeding from our vagina I'm told.

You hold it well doctor.

Well, what took you so long to get care? Your blood level is down to a hemoglobin of 6. That's not good.

I'm not surprised.

Let me put my fingers inside, and . . .yes that's good, spread your legs. . . God Damn. You didn't have to drip on my gown, I just changed it! Oh. There's a thing in there. Hm . . . quite a thing.

A thing, doctor?

Yes. If it's a tumor it could be cancer and you could die.

Really?

Yes! You women are something else! You wait and wait and wait and then at the last minute you come in and expect us to act like gods. '*Heal my cancer, Oh god in white.*'

Are you sure it's cancer?

Of course not. You'll need a CT Scan and a workup and an examination by a gynecologist.

So when do we begin?

Probably after 7:00 AM when the next shift comes on. I'm pooped. I've been taking care of infected ears all night. We'll start an IV and have the AM doc see you. Good luck. Oh, by the way, are you Catholic because I can get the Father to give you Last Rites. He's in the next booth right now. And I'll tell the nurse to get another Tampax.

Doctor walks out muttering, "Dumb old broad! Nearly bleeds to death from a vaginal tumor and waits forever to seek care!"

CURTAIN FALLS

ANNOUNCER: And so ends THE EPIC OF ELOISE, brought to you by the Drama Department of Lesser Arcana Productions. We hope you enjoyed this horror story. Is it true? I'm ashamed to admit that the individuals who are most likely to deny what I have written here are the very health professionals who are closest to the truth of our little play. You might want to explore the chance that this is entirely a fantasy. Just remember that you may have to live with your rationalizations if it happens to you.

THE END

---

In spite of all of this It's surprising how much optimism has entered the field of cancer research in the last few years. Talking of cures (!) is not out of the question any longer!

In addition we may be learning how to dodge the issue in many cases. For instance cervical cancer is the second most common form of cancer in women. Recent evidence reinforces the old suspicion that it's probably a venereal disease! There are at least 35 types of Human Papilloma Virus (HPV). Ten types cause genital warts and 25 types are now found linked to cervical cancer.

The smoking gun was the HPV DNA found in 95 percent of the tumors surveyed in over a thousand women in 22 countries. Specifically HPV 16 was found to accompany over half of the cancers in the study, three others were there for another 30 percent, and the remainder entrained lesser numbers. These HPV types manufacture proteins which are presumed to cause tumors. Cervical cancer is the second most common form of cancer worldwide, striking about 500,000 women annually, with 8 out of 10 cases in the developing world.

People are beginning to talk of possible vaccines for HPV and thus possibly preventing, or even curing, cervical cancer.

Here's a magic word for you: "*methylation*". That's what turns your genes off, and an error can cause real trouble. Consider a benign example first, the gene for hemoglobin. Every cell has it. Only red blood cells need it. The "*promoter*' region of the gene is methylated (turned off) in all except red blood cells.

It's not just mutation we need to worry about. What if a tumor suppresser gene was accidentally methylated? Right. Cancer!

You can also turn genes back on, at least in cell cultures, so there is a dream that cancer can be cured with drugs, after more research. Several biotech companies are beginning to explore this approach. For more on cancer and its prevention see my remarks on nutrients in chapter 20.

The entire human genome may well be sequenced by about the time you read this. Fine tuning, racial sorting, and the usual frightening implications, are next. Let us not forget that with genetics in the news, the eugenicists can not be far behind, so we can look forward to rabid racism. Everything has become political today, including your DNA.

If someone gets your DNA they know all about you. The national data bases can only get bigger. The idea of privacy seems to be pretty much dead. Freedom and repression are both going to have to be redefined by our grandchildren. More on cancer in Chapters 6 and 17.

# 14

## AIDS - The New Plague

In the 19th. century a wise man said that "*physicians and politicians resemble one another in this respect, that one defends the constitution, and the other destroys it.*" I think I'll just let that one lie there till it goes off.

We are told, and may even believe, that we are drinking safe, clean, proper water. We believe we are breathing somewhat nearly OK air. We believe we are living in freedom from epidemics. So far it's been true enough, but the flow across our borders, and the little critters who bite, bring several cases every year of cholera, and even on one occasion dreaded Ebola, to our shores. Every intervention may disturb another delicate balance.

Ground dwelling rodents, prairie dogs and others, as well as family pets, especially cats, have helped build a pool of potential plague infection spread by fleas in the American Southwest, primarily in New Mexico, Arizona, Colorado, and California. I'm talking about Bubonic Plague here folks, the Black Death! We seem to be in no immediate danger but in the last 50 years there have been 400 cases of Bubonic Plague in the United States!

A lot of foodborne and waterborne infection is going unnoticed and undetected. We become convinced of our untouchability in America, and environmental hazards are ignored and unaddressed.

This leaves us with a quiet way to cut the budget, trim the staff, destroy morale and motivation among the rapid response teams, and get re-elected. **It gives us an excuse to fire those who most deeply care.** We ignore our water even when it smells of parasites and dissolved industrial waste. Malignant neglect is everywhere. There is no malignant neglect of the dollar. Don't worry - be happy!

And guys, don't lick your balls before hitting them at the golf course. There may be harmful pesticide residues on them, according to a British sports magazine. Sorry about that.

We barely notice that in the last 10 years acute infections have turned into chronic infections, Tuberculosis is back, but we largely ignore it, although the World Health Organization (WHO) reports that an epidemic of "*new-tuberculosis*" raging in Russia has now spread to Scandinavia. The Russian rate of infection is more than nine times that in the U.S. Tuberculosis already kills three million people worldwide each year, three times as many as die from HIV. WHO scientific officer, Chris Dye, characterizes current U.S. containment efforts as "*embryonic*". Malaria and dengue, usually considered tropical diseases, are also moving ever closer to our borders as global warming begins.

The danger from the new, as well as the re-emerging old, isn't lessened by increasingly useless antibiotics. We are reversing our progress from Pasteur until today.

A recent report from the World Health Organization warns that the spread of untreatable forms of malaria and tuberculosis and the emergence of killers like AIDS and Ebola threaten us.

More than one million people died of AIDS in 1995. About 20 million are infected, according to WHO. Diseases that have been around for centuries are cropping up in incurable strains. Even AIDS apparently crossed over from monkeys to humans sometime before World War II. More than 17 million people die every year from infectious diseases. "We are standing on the brink of a global crisis in infectious diseases," said the Director-General of WHO, Dr. Hiroshi Nakajima.

While we are ignoring all of this, we find the Mod Med Biz available on any stock exchange, if not in every home. How could that HIV outbreak downtown matter, to those of us in Hacienda Heights? Our doctors seem to have lost their vision, from so much peering at the bottom line perhaps. We are losing well qualified health care professionals and gaining well qualified merchants, marketers, accountants, CEO's. Does God hide in the details of the Quarterly Report or the Dow averages?

Congress decides this is a good time to gut the funding for the National Center for Injury Prevention and Control. You are noticing who is supporting this sort of thing I hope. The coming election may be bad for your health.

Sexual behavior spreads the old diseases once again, hantavirus comes from a house mouse, travel and trade bring more than computers with the tide, and we need to spend more on the exploration of space. The Centers for Disease Control (CDC) say, "*The present cost of antibiotic resistance in the United States is 30 billion dollars a year, and growing daily.*" More space is between the legislators ears than near the moons of Jupiter.

Be afraid. There is a new devil out there. Even the Hollywood screen writers have heard, and they are almost as slow as politicians to understand the world we are living in. You might like to know a bit about Ebola.

Ebola is not alone. In our mad rush to turn Eden into a parking lot, we're digging up all kinds of nasty organisms which have been there quietly all along. We're building dams and breeding mosquitoes. Hospitals in tropical countries aren't quite State-of-the-Art yet, and it would help if they could afford to change the bedding after the patient dies.

A common thread that runs through all the known (!) Ebola epidemics is poverty and abysmal medical facilities. Africa is not the only place suffering from these problems! Recently someone noticed that the symptoms of the plague, that decimated ancient Athens and changed the course of history, sounds very much like an early outbreak of Ebola. Be very afraid!

Things are escaping into the world, i.e. they "*come to light when environmental conditions change*", and the next intercontinental jet is scheduled to arrive just in time to carry them to Kansas City. The CDC in Atlanta are having a harder time keeping up.

At the moment the subject is hemorrhagic fever viruses. I won't go into details but we're talking about a lot of blood and messy death here:

Hemorrhagic fever viruses come in at least four flavors. The (1) *flaviviruses* have been known the longest (among them is the Amaril virus responsible for yellow fever, and dengue), (2) *arenaviruses*

(Guanarito, Machupo, Junin, Lassa, and Sabia), (3) *bunyaviruses* (the "*hantaviruses*") much in the news. Non fatal Puumala, and Sin Nombre are both bunyaviruses. And (4) the most dangerous member of the hemorrhagic fever family, the *filoviruses* (Marburg, Ebola!).

All the arenaviruses and bunyaviruses circulate naturally and generally non-lethally in various populations of animals which serve as the reservoirs for human epidemics. Rodents don't show symptoms but drop large quantities of feces and urine along their dusty trails. This all blows in the wind kicked up by our bulldozers and helicopters. We don't know yet how the filoviruses get around. Generally all the hemorrhagic fever viruses mutate a lot and genetically re-combine with each other as well, which is really scary.

It helps to have a scholarly name for death. In the case of hemorrhagic fever viruses the words are "*emerging pathogens*". In the last 10 years we've been getting better at finding emerging pathogens. It took only 8 days to identify the bunyavirus called Sin Nombre. Feel better?

Many of these diseases are so hazardous they cannot be handled except in laboratories that conform to very strict safety requirements. It is dangerous to handle infected monkeys, yet the viruses cannot be studied in more common laboratory animals such as rats, because these creatures do not become ill when infected.

Research on microbes that are found primarily in developing countries has for many years been poorly funded. Were Ebola, or any hemorrhagic fever virus, to acquire genetic characteristics suitable for airborne transmission, an outbreak of disease anywhere would pose a threat to all humanity.

It begins to look as though God has prepared His own solution to our population problems, if we don't soon succeed in solving them ourselves. We won't.

---

## LE BAISER DE LE FE

*an opera-lite*

*by*

*Gershon Prasinus and Giuseppe Verdi*

ANNOUNCER: It's time for one more of the million stories from the city. It's time for LE BAISER DE LE FE, or Hippocrates Bound, an opera-lite in three scenes, one interlude, and two settings, with libretto by Gershon Prasinus and music by Giuseppe Verdi. The action takes place in The Green and Greene Ecological Hospital and Holistic Clinic (GGEHHC), situated like an emerald in the green belt of Green Pernt, New York.

Before the curtain rises we see a sample of one of Dr. Yoo's (not his real name) television commercials on the screen above the stage: Happily playing children are seen behind the sincere face of an actor who looks very much like a middle aged Walter Cronkite in a white lab coat, stethoscope draped plonkingly from his pocket. He removes his glasses, leans forward, and speaks:

"*In these times of impersonal managed care and HMO disinterest, you need to be interested in a doctor interested in you. Let me tell you of doctor Lovehart Yoo. He lives in your community. His children go to the same schools as your children. He shops at the same Save-U Mart you do. Doctor Yoo cares! His telephone number is 555-3825. In the tradition of Hippocrates, Dr. Yoo places the person first, not HMO rules, or money matters. What matters to Dr. Yoo is you. Call 555-3825. Whatever your pain or suffering, Yoo steps into your moccasins and walks a mile with you. Dr. Yoo feels the issues that concern you, ponders them, connects with you in a caring fashion. That's 555-3825. There is no therapy without love between healer and healee.* (music rises to a climax as the choir sings, "*Do Yoo Care? He do! 555-3825*" - music segues into Verdi's overture to Le Baiser de le Fe.)

- and the curtain rises on Scene 1. We are in Dr. Yoo's waiting room. There are a great many green vinyl plants arranged tastefully on the walls, floor, and hanging from the ceiling. The early afternoon sun shines brightly in through a wall of glass, casting leaf shadows on the wall.

John Doe enters the waiting room just behind another patient who looks a great deal like Desmond Tutu, the South African cleric. The wall clock says exactly 1:58 PM. The reception window is closed. They sit down. Doe is almost sure it is Bishop Tutu. No one else is present. John Doe waits. The window does not open. Exactly four minutes later he turns to Father Tutu and sings:

(JOHN DOE, COUNTERTENOR) Maybe my watch is wrong. Am I right? Have you been here from two to 2:00 to 2:00 two too, Tutu?

The good bishop says nothing, stands, and moves to the other end of the waiting room.

Doe goes over and knocks on the window. Rose (SOPRANO) opens the sliding window, revealing a card with the Deep Ecology Manifesto on it, and sings:

My name is Rose. You may call me Rose. What?

I'm John Doe, Rose. I have a 1:45 PM appointment?

You do?

Yes. I heard about you on TV and called the next day.

Oh let's see. I have a John Doo. Perhaps someone misspelled your name?

I guess.

Do you have insurance?

Yes.

Well? Where is your card, hon?

You need a card, dear?"

While you're at it, fill out these forms.

(Doe, digging through wallet, finds Green Shield card) Is this what you want?

Yes. Is that all you have?

I guess.

(RECEPTIONIST - sings the Flying Standards aria:)

Well I hope it covers everything.
You know you're responsible for the bill.
We never let the insurance company set our fees.
That "usual and standard community practice" doesn't fly here.
You pay what we bill.
Let's get the form filled out.

(John Doe sits down and goes to work. The window closes. He finishes and waits in the bright sunlight.)

(ANNOUNCER) And so the curtain falls on the first scene of LE BAISER DE LE FE by Prasinus and Verdi. In just a moment, after a few words from our author, we will return for The Interlude.

---

One quarter of central Africa will die of AIDS if things continue on as they are! It only took 56 patriots to sign the Declaration of Independence.

Can I, can you, remain unconcerned in the face of an epidemic that will surely kill millions of innocent people? I wonder if your family doctor, any health giving human being, any government worthy of the name, can do so. AIDS is not a judgment from heaven. We have time to recognize the face of our brothers and our sisters before they die. My mother is never wrong, and it is she who says, "*Never waste good agony.*"

A healthy lifestyle may extend the life of HIV positive people and may delay the onset of AIDS in people found HIV positive. Most of the Americans suffering from AIDS have no money for a "*healthy lifestyle*" or the new medications so much in the news. Who is to pay for a healthy "lifestyle" for the millions of HIV positive Africans soon to die?

HIV positive smokers will progress to full blown AIDS at twice the rate of nonsmokers. Consumption of alcohol was found to speed the AIDS onset and scientists now tell us that alcohol in fact reduces immunity seriously. And so we learn of complicities within complicities and once again see ourselves in the mirror of history.

Uncircumcised African men are particularly susceptible to AIDS.[1] The stress level in HIV infection is becoming an issue. Stress may alter natural killer cell counts and cytotoxic T-cells in HIV infected patients. The psychiatric interview is becoming important. Our dry as dust academic emotional indicators have difficulty with all this.

Vitamin E and beta carotene appear to be safe and effective in delaying the progression of HIV infection to clinical AIDS, decreasing symptoms associated with the illness, and perhaps even contributing to long term survival.

AIDS patients have a progressive decrease in antioxidant levels as the disease worsens. Most AIDS and HIV infected patients studied were consuming less than half the RDA (!) for vitamin E. Researchers concluded that intake of antioxidants at levels considerably above RDA is needed to maintain adequate blood nutrient status in HIV positive patients.

In one study, over 90 percent of HIV infected patients who ingested a combination of vitamins daily, experienced a 2 year survival rate showing no evidence of disease progression. AIDS patients given 60 mg per day of beta carotene had apparent recovery from night sweating, fever, diarrhea, and weight loss and a significantly increased total white blood cell count.

We're nibbling away at AIDS. Lowered white and red blood cell counts brought on by chemotherapy and high-dose radiation can be controlled by drugs. Low platelet counts will soon be fought with an alphabet drug called "*MGDF*" if early studies bear fruit, and dangerous blood transfusions may not be needed as often. It is sometimes the small incremental improvements that help the most in our efforts to control disease.

Supplementing the protection of condoms against the spread of AIDS, a new vaginal gel containing "*PMPA*," being studied at the

National Institute of Infectious Diseases, seems to be more effective than "*non-oxynol-9*" in early trials with monkeys. It is possible it might even be effective after intercourse. Many medicines look impressive in monkeys but fail with people.

A couple of years ago, a study in North Carolina showed that AZT given to pregnant women and their newborns prevented AIDS in a significant number of the infants. How can we measure the joy of the mothers of that "*significant number*" of healthy babies?

As of this writing there are 11 approved drugs used in AIDS therapy, and 25 drugs available for related conditions with the number going up almost monthly. That's probably good news if you're a rich American, but nobody knows how good. The drugs include good old toxic zidovudine (AZT), plus lamivudine (3TC) and indinavir (trade named Crixivan - where do they get these names). AZT and 3TC are "*reverse transcriptase inhibitors*" (nucleoside analogs), and hit the virus earlier, at a different point in its reproductive cycle. Then there is a group of reverse transcriptase inhibitors which are *non*nucleoside analogues. Nevirapine (Viramune) is in this group.

More treatment strategies are coming, involving such numbers as ABT-378, PNU-140690 as well as hydroxyurea, an old and *inexpensive* (!) drug adapted for indirect use against HIV.

There may also be ALX40-4C against several strains of HIV. It seems to prevent the HIV virus from entering the "CD4 lymphocytes", the body's immune system cells which are the main target of HIV and responsible for immune system collapse when depleted. ALX40-4C worked especially well in laboratory tests against those strains of HIV that cause the most trouble, and it may soon join our arsenal of drugs effective in some way against HIV.

In the absence of a cure, the hope is that the virus's reproduction can be slowed down. This would prevent the rapid mutation rate that has caused us so much trouble, and allow our immune system to remain intact longer. If HIV does not become resistant to the drugs, and they can be given safely for many years, AIDS can be treated successfully as a chronic disease.

Antioxidants combined with the new drugs may have therapeutic benefits and may allow drugs to be used in lower doses thus limiting toxicity and decreasing production of drug resistant HIV strains.

The newest addition to the list of useable drugs will cost 7,000 dollars a year, and that's only one drug. There are hundreds of possible combinations of various drugs in use. Combination anti-HIV therapy costs $12,000 to $18,000 a year, and the many other medications that patients with advanced AIDS may need for related conditions could raise the bill to $70,000 a year! In addition, as many as 20 percent of HIV-positive patients fail drug therapy because they cannot tolerate the side effects.

This is not a trivial concern. Side effects can include nausea, diarrhea, pancreatic or mouth inflammation, peripheral neuropathy, headache, anemia, low white blood cell counts, weakness, insomnia, rash, hepatitis, kidney stones, abnormal distribution of fat, blurred vision, dizziness, and elevated triglyceride or cholesterol levels, among many others only bearable when you consider the alternative.

These prices are supposed to allow the drug companies to recoup the cost of their development, After the patent expires, other companies can make generic versions of the same drugs and charge as little as they want, in order to compete. Drug maker Bristol-Myers Squibb and other drug companies recently attempted to get Congress to extend their monopolies on best selling brand name drugs, such as the cancer treatment Taxol and the allergy medicine Claritin.

I suppose this is as good a place as any other to mention something that may save you a lot of money when it's pill time. Pricing of medications is based on subtle and arcane equations that do not always mirror the quantity you are getting. You can sometimes buy the double size pill for very little more than the one you were prescribed. Pay just a bit more and break the pills in half! You can sometimes save nearly half the cost. The only thing you need to keep in mind is that the coating on some pills may have a function such as protecting your stomach, and of course you shouldn't open capsules. You can crack most pills by hand. If not, there are $4.00 pill splitters available at the pharmacy.

Despite evolving evidence that antioxidants and other nutrients are effective, financial support for nutritional therapies is largely unavailable until patients develop full blown AIDS, and by then the potential benefits are diminished.

We still don't know what the proper dosage balance should be. We don't know how long each chemical will be useful in the patient. And most important we don't yet know how the HMO's and the insurance companies, are going to respond to all this. I'm lying - that's "*lawyer talk*". Of course we know how the HMO's and the insurance companies are going to respond to all this.

It is quite clear that we need more and better funded research immediately!

We have a lethal triage taking shape in our health care system. I wonder if it will be as easy to find the money to treat an AIDS patient who is 61 years old as it will be to treat one who is 31 - or 11! And I think it's safe to say that it will be too long before these drugs are available for the prostitutes of Nairobi.

A controversial report has been published stating that a type of HIV virus now mostly confined to Africa and Asia is soon to reach our shores. The new strain spreads very quickly through heterosexual populations! That should help wake us up. So far there are at least eleven strains of HIV, within two major types, M and O, and counting. They differ from each other in their structure. They also differ in their geographical distribution and perhaps in their mode of attack.

What will not be explained is why, with all the promises, and all the numbers and abbreviations, our government (It is **our** government remember?) makes no significant investment to gain the secrets of the most devious and frightening health threat since the Black Death of the Middle Ages (!), the AIDS virus.

---

## LE BAISER DE LE FE

ANNOUNCER: In Scene 1 of LE BAISER DE LE FE: or Hippocrates Bound, we left our hero, John Doe, almost entirely alone in the sunlight filled waiting room of The GGEHHC, situated like an emerald in the green belt of Green Pernt, New York. The Interlude takes place in front of the lowered curtain. Ten minutes after finishing his paper work, John Doe knocks on the receptionists window:

(ROSE) What?

Here are the forms, Rose.

Oh yes. Let's see, you didn't put down your license plate number or your social security number! What are they?

Why?

I have to protect Doctor Yoo from insurance fraud. You could be someone else!

If I was someone else, I'd be someplace else, and not here. You don't sound very loving to me!

(disdainfully) Your numbers please?

(Doe sings them melodiously)

Now come into the examination room please. (She swiftly walks out of sight behind the curtain. John Doe has no idea where she went. She comes back.) Please Mr. Doo. We can't waste time can we? Put on that lascivious paper gown and sit on the table.

(They disappear behind the curtain and The Interlude of LE BAISER DE LE FE comes to an end. The Transition music combines elements of a gavotte, a gallope, and a trotte.) ANNOUNCER: In just a moment, after a few words from our author, we will return for Scene Two in which we learn what this is all about. (The trotte gavotte continues.)

---

It is said, "*It is better to die on your feet than to live on your knees.*" I like another version better, "*Live, even fight, on your knees until you can rise up, because they win if you die on your feet.*" You fight this battle with scientific research.

One of the heart aches produced by more conservative research into possible vaccines for HIV is that antibodies produced are often directed at a part of the virus' envelope that is not on the exterior, but hidden in the interior of the virus. As a result, even if the antibodies are circulating in a person's blood, they have no effect because their target is hidden.

■ 1.) Which brings me to a new focus. Dr. Jonas Salk developed another vaccine before he died, a vaccine which he believed might well prevent a person from catching and developing the AIDS virus and its disease, as he pointed out when he was a guest on my radio program. This vaccine is made from a live HIV virus, which is first treated to a massive dose of gamma radiation, which Dr. Salk tells us, kills whatever life a virus may be said to have.[1]

The vaccine is then injected into a human as is any other, flu, polio, measles, tetanus, pneumonia - and there you have it. As basic and fundamental an idea as Dr. Jenner's, whose vaccine went on to eradicate smallpox from planet earth.

Dr. Salk took his own vaccine, but you are not allowed to have it. You see, a "*reputable minority*" raised the question, "*What if but one in one million HIV viruses was not dead?*" Good question, as Dr. Salk himself had reason to remember. An early batch of the Salk polio vaccine inadvertently gave polio to 100 children, and yes; it is controversial. In these days, controversy usually becomes part of the problem, although Pasteur would have understood just as well, in those days.

This controversy, like most, is born of fear. Dr. Salk pointed out that no living molecule can survive that potent a blast of gamma radiation. Keeping the cockroach in mind at all times, there are those who disagree.

We must learn the first lesson of life, which is to control our own smoke, prejudice included, and not inflict our personal fear or morbidness on others. The chances of getting AIDS for certain groups of homosexuals and drug abusers are a whole lot more than one in a million. The rest of us can certainly learn to juggle million-to-one odds for ourselves, if anyone would ever level with us, which isn't very likely.

Aside from the small problem raised by the "reputable minority", the practical issue which blocks your seeing this vaccine is that the company which agreed to produce it for world usage, can't get medical product liability insurance, or malpractice insurance, for any price. Be sure to consult your law care professional.

If they went ahead anyway, you know in your bones that the very next day there would be platoons of attorneys, with that generic client, in association with those generic expert-witness medical doctors, all of equally marvelous moral fiber, all of whom would bring a devastating product liability or medical malpractice case ("*...did maliciously, willfully, and with negligence.....this poor victim who with trust and innocence...*") which would entangle all remaining freedom to act in such degree as to bankrupt even Novartis, and Hoffmann-La Roche combined, overnight. That is the issue isn't it?

In parts of Black Africa nearly 25 percent of the population, men, women, and children, is HIV-positive as a result of heterosexual transmission of the virus. As these individuals develop full blown AIDS, we will see many more millions of deaths result. Dr. Salk's million to one odds look better and better for those not yet infected (this is not a cure), even if the "*reputable minority*" is right.

The United States government, under President Ford, purchased the swine flu vaccine and gave it to every interested doctor in

America, to be administered free to their patients, with legal protection for any liability claims. The lethal flu never materialized, thereby proving the lawyers were right. Right?

It's the only time something like that has ever happened, and you can be sure it will never happen again, AIDS vaccine notwithstanding. The governments of the world could legislate away liability, and in the absence of that kind of sense, they could go the swine flu route. Don't they know this is a major world life and death issue? Of course they do. Don't they care? No, they don't! They think it's only Black Africans, gays and dope addicts. But it's already a lot more than that! I hope we are never faced with an Ebola epidemic!

- 2.) (read these carefully) There was a report in The Lancet in which a randomized trial in six communities in rural areas of Tanzania showed that treatment of sexually transmitted diseases like syphilis and gonorrhea reduced the incidence of HIV infection by about 40 percent, for the first time showing that controlling sexually transmitted diseases also seemed to control HIV.

- 3.) Henry Heimlich has another maneuver for us. Considering how the medical establishment fought his original idea, maybe we should do more research on his current one.[3]

  In 1987 he asked the Centers for Disease Control for some malaria infected blood. Heimlich thinks he has a cure (!) for AIDS that doesn't involve drugs, needs to be administered only once, and would last a lifetime. No one is listening of course. He was refused and rebuffed in print as you might expect. He is now working in China and has opened a research clinic in Mexico where his ideas are available to the public.

  Don't go away yet, there's some historical precedent. Since 1917 when Dr. Wagner-Juaregg introduced the concept, for which he got the Nobel Prize in 1927, malaria therapy has been the treatment of choice for syphilis of the brain, and is still used for that disease when antibiotics fail.

What's happening here? It's the fever of malaria of course, but also various “cytokines” (tumor necrosis factor, interferons, interleukins) stimulated by malaria which may “*kick start*” the immune system. Malaria therapy involves giving an individual a case of malaria, letting the fever continue for about three weeks, and then curing the malaria. According to Wren MacCager, tens of thousands of patients have been cured of neurosyphilis in this manner, and all cases of induced therapeutic malaria since 1917 have been cured in their turn.

The danger lies in giving a potentially fatal disease to someone who already has no ability to fight infection. However, a study of 112 children in Africa showed that approximately one-third of the children also had AIDS. Later one-third of the AIDS-only infected children died, but *none* (!) of those also infected with malaria died.

In addition, a study conducted by researchers from the University of Nebraska in conjunction with a Navy medical research unit, identified malarial regions in Africa where AIDS does not exist! The population of those regions did however possess antibodies to AIDS. Also there are individual cases (“*anecdotal evidence*”) where Heimlich's ideas have been born out.

■ 4.) Over the past ten years 36 different AIDS vaccines have been injected into more than 2,000 people. We don't know whether they work or not with such small samples. Now similar vaccines made by biotech companies are being given a large scale trial.[2] They will be tried on two different strains of HIV rampant in Thailand, including a new and extremely dangerous one. Ninety percent of HIV infected Thais are heterosexual! Over 100,000 Thais are dying annually of AIDS and the rate will keep climbing unless something can be done. Because both of these vaccines only use part of the HIV virus, it will be impossible for them to cause AIDS. Other countries and other vaccine tests may follow.

- 5.) There is even a minority opinion that AIDS as a distinct disease does not exist. Prof. Peter Duesberg of UC Berkeley has been saying for 10 years that the HIV virus is a harmless hitchhiker in the blood of thousands of people whose immune systems have been ruined by environmental poisons, drugs, and behavior.

There are various other vaccine strategies now under study, not always with human subjects. Some potential vaccines elicit anti-HIV antibodies, some elicit cellular responses, and some combine approaches.

Does this mean that we are close to having a cure for AIDS? ***No!*** As I said at the beginning of this speculation, we need more research, but AIDS is too destructive and the potential for disaster is too high, to allow any ideas, no matter how controversial they may seem, to be buried by "*standard*" or "*orthodox*" thinking. Full flexibility is called for in times of maximum tension and danger. We may be ignoring Louis Pasteur once again. Let us acquit ourselves with honor this time.

---

## LE BAISER DE LE FE

ANNOUNCER: In Scene 2 of LE BAISER DE LE FE: or Hippocrates Bound, by Prasinus and Verdi, we find our hero, John Doe, in the examination room of The GGEHHC, situated like an emerald in the green belt of Green Pernt, New York. Later afternoon sunlight pours through the green privacy screen onto John Doe, dressed in a green paper gown, stickily sitting on a green paper covered table. A nurse is standing by. Dr. Yoo (baritone) enters and sings:

Hello. You're Dao?

I'm Doe, Yoo, or Dao to you.

(Dr. Lovehart Yoo looks at paper in green folder:) I see. Chinese I guess. You look Caucasian to me, Johnny.

No, no. I'm Tibetan, Lovehart. It's been in the family for years.

Hm. (sung with fervor.)

What's the trouble John? Asthma? A sore throat?

(John Doe sings the Great White Spot aria:)
I don't know, Yoo.
I'm too tired for a 24 year old.
I'm losing weight, and
Sweating when I shouldn't be.
I have these white spots
On my tongue,
And when I cut myself it takes forever to heal.
I get sore throat
After sore throat.
I know I'm sick.
I don't know, doctor Yoo!

DOCTOR YOO: Well. OK. Have you ever had Hepatitis, or Mononucleosis John?

No. I did have Herpes, Lovehart.

Did your lip swell.

(music goes to minor key, ominous rumble from the drums:) No. I had ulcers on my penis.

Oh, you had a sexually transmitted disease Mister Dao?

If you want to call it that I guess.

Well you ought to know better. Lot's of loose young women with a lot of stuff out there.

(the drums are back, along with a muttering from the violins:) Well, sir. I don't get it on with women. You know, like I'm gay.

(Dr. Yoo is aghast:) Gay? Gad, Dao! Why would you want to be that?

I guess God made me that way.

But it's a sin! You have a hell of a problem. What do you do? Oral?

Anal.

My God! And you expect to be well?

Well I don't know what to expect, but I'm sick right now.

Well I'll just do a checkup. Bend over. (Puts on two pairs of latex gloves, one on top of the other. Takes three seconds for the checkup. Sings to nurse:)
Take a blood test of Dao.
Run a blood sugar test of Dao.
Check the cholesterol of Dao.
Oh, Dao!
And do an HIV test of Dao. (observe all repeats)

(Doctor leaves room, Nurse dons three pairs of latex gloves, takes blood samples, and leaves.)

More trotte gavotte signals the passage of 15 minutes. The vinyl plants grow. Doctor Yoo returns:) Mr. Dao, your spot HIV test is positive.

What does that mean? (the orchestra is going into ominous fits by this time.)

Mister John Dao, you're in the wrong place. I don't treat AIDS. I suggest you go to one of those doctors who treat people like you.

Like me? Do I have AIDS?

Yes, it's likely.

You mean I could die?

Well that's something you should have thought about before committing your dirty acts, not after, isn't it?

What are you going to do to help me, Doctor Yoo?

Go see someone else. AIDS was sent by God.

Is this the love therapy you advertise?"

I'm interested in normal people, not perverts. Go get dressed. (Doctor exits.)

ANNOUNCER: And so the curtain falls on the second scene of LE BAISER DE LE FE, the opera-lite by Prasinus and Verdi. In just a moment, after a few words from our author, we will return for the third and final scene of our one-act opera.

---

"*Fix reason firmly in her seat,*" wrote Thomas Jefferson, "*and call on her tribunal for every fact, every opinion.*" The trial attorneys, and the legislators have made it clear what they want. All they need to know from you is what you won't stand for. Righteous and constructive anger is good for the soul if it brings out the best in us, and saves the lives of the rest of us!

It is the obligation of every medical doctor, of every person who in any way calls him or herself a member of the healing arts, of every social scientist, not to speak of the White House, the halls of the Health and Human Services Department, the National Institutes of Health, the Centers For Disease Control, the Congress, or even the state capitols, to see that the imperative investment in AIDS research is made, and made "with all deliberate speed." The tragedy in such a phrase however is that even such words fix no early or inescapable date for compliance. We seem to have no such doubts for the date of our income tax.

There really is a significantly frightening major epidemic out there. HIV is a viral attack well entrenched in the larger social structure, and a syndrome well on its way to tearing great holes in certain other cultures. The only reason you don't hear as much about this today is that the new medications have persuaded the media that the problem is solved. It is not.

A diagnosis as dramatic as AIDS or cancer is one of the most shattering life problems a person needs to face. A person with this diagnosis instantly disconnects from society, withdraws, weakens, may consider suicide. The physician may be looking at a blood cell count, not the depression of the patient, which is a combination of fear, anger, and guilt, which no one is really paying attention to.

A diagnosis of AIDS immediately elicits the same symptoms as those suffered by the soldier in battle. The patients panic, they vomit, they get diarrhea, they hyperventilate, they get dizzy, they get cardiac rhythm problems and could have themselves a good coronary. I wonder if there are any atheists with AIDS?

I have learned well how a label diagnosis can break a human heart, and does! As long as we are alive, we must never forget that we have the ability to exercise free will. A mind that has chosen to survive has many choices. We are capable of creating the world brick by brick. Every brick of self esteem and faith builds yet more of our spiritual, psychological and physiological defense. Our immune cells have the ability to turn disease into "*good luck.*"

"*Why talk to me so loftily of purification and healing,*" says the AIDS patient, "*the experts say otherwise.*" The experts are wrong, say I. Weak, frightened, and tired, we are robbed at our lowest point of hope and faith, by so called experts. There are no experts in the art of life!

We walk the narrow bridge between healing and illness, life and death, suffering and ease, knowledge and ignorance, and the spiritual dimensions of life can shift the balance in the right direction.

Believing only "*what we already know*" doomed the leper until the courts freed him from the devil, and science cured him.

There's a bias out there about people who suffer AIDS. Who, in the Mod Med Biz, gives a damn? Where can our family turn if they do give a damn? They may lose the ability to communicate with you. They may not even know how to say goodbye!

We have to try to say something to people in their loneliness that can offer some realistic encouragement. They can really do something about their problem, even if it is only to cherish the time and love they have left.

As the moment of death approaches, one takes a good long look at one's entire life, and what one's expectations might have been, and how it will not happen! This is painful.

What would you do if the disease were of such a nature that you couldn't even talk about it. What if you were silenced, because successful communication in your case would entail judgments, biases, prejudices, in others?

A sense of guilt is one of the worst gifts we have given to AIDS patients. If we could learn new ways of thinking, their viruses would not kill them so easily. The emotions, sad states, mad states, are critical to the function of immunity, and immunity is critical to almost every illness you can think of.

We respond emotionally to the disease, and we respond to the emotion, in feedback. Any engineer can tell you that this is an excellent way to go out of control. Most of us have experienced feedback in public address systems or on the air. It is a squeal of outraged electrons, a little like the squeal of sick, outraged, and frightened people.

# LE BAISER DE LE FE

ANNOUNCER: The curtain rises on Scene 3 of LE BAISER DE LE FE, or Hippocrates Bound, an opera-lite in three scenes, one interlude, and two settings, with libretto by Gershon Prasinus and music by Giuseppe Verdi. The action takes place in The GGEHHC, situated like an emerald in the green belt of Green Pernt, New York. We are back in Dr. Yoo's waiting room. The late afternoon sun seems to be under a cloud. It looks like rain. The other patient in the waiting room, wearing a clerical collar, is being strangled by a vinyl Ficus benjamina

(John Doe is walking out through the reception area. The window slams open and Rose sings:

Yoo hoo Doo, just a moment!

What?

That will be 300 dollars.

For what?

You've got some nerve mister. You took up a full hour of doc's time!

Firstly lady, he took up a full hour of my time, between ignoring me, insuring me, photocopying me, insulting me, and sticking me. He did nothing for me in the end, as it were. He sent me off somewhere else.

Well that's what he gets paid for. We don't sell tires at GGEHHC. If he sent you somewhere that's good medical advice.

Lady, you don't want a check from me. I just learned that the AIDS virus gets carried in ink. You might catch it from touching my check.

Oh! Well, in that case, give me a credit card number. You don't have to sign. Could you step back from the window please?

No I don't have a credit card. Send me a bill, hon. (John Doe holds out his hand to shake hands. Rose recoils.)

Good bye, Mr. Doo.

No return visit? Love certainly abounds here, Rose. Maybe I ought to refer some of my gay friends.

I'm sorry. We don't have any open appointments for at least seven months. Goodbye. (Slams window shut. Set revolves. Mary turns to female typist, now in view, and sings:)

That fag out there has some nerve, coming in to our office. Imagine it! He has AIDS! I'm not going to catch AIDS that way. We always have to worry about these sex diseases!

(contralto typist sings:) Don't worry Rosey. When you and I get it on, there's no way we can catch AIDS. My dildo doesn't spit, remember?

ANNOUNCER: And so the curtain falls on the third and final scene of LE BAISER DE LE FE, or Hippocrates Bound, an opera-lite in three scenes, one interlude, and two settings, with libretto by Gershon Prasinus and music by Giuseppe Verdi. The action took place in The Green and Greene Ecological Hospital and Holistic Clinic, situated like an emerald in the green belt of Green Pernt, New York. Now we return to our author:

THE END

We seldom realize that this is a very tough country to live in. The middle and upper classes always do well in any country, but if you're homeless or get AIDS, it's tough dude! It makes civilization a bit gummy, shallow, easily fractured, doesn't it? How can this promote healing in someone who needs a generally dramatic support system?

This is one of the reasons I am pointing so heavily to the spiritual in this book. It's at the base of alcoholics anonymous, drug withdrawal programs, hospices, and halfway houses of all kinds. Why is it not also the basis of officially offered AIDS therapy?

The diagnosis of AIDS may lead to swift death, or no effects for 10 years. Fatalities go down during periods of high challenge or in individuals expecting an event such as the birth of a child. Chinese death rates peak after their New Year. The emotional flux clearly influences the level of wellness or illness we experience. A given situation may empower some people and panic others.

The entire range of a person's well being and self orientation changes with the simple application of a label. Tell someone they have Alzheimer's Disease and they'll do far worse than if you tell them they have a little memory loss, "*so write things down and carry a memory pad with you.*"

As physicians we usually do not notice how much grief, sorrow, loss, anger, fear, anxiety, guilt, are building up in any illness. In breast cancer cases, suppression leads to more metastases. How can we learn how to turn scared into sacred?

The Buddhists teach us that we can become enlightened despite our pain. There's a crucial point of understanding that is missing in the objective scientific view of human suffering and disease, no matter how expert the opinion. The patient often senses this lack of linkage and may feel powerless and seriously depressed.

Need I remind us that native American traditional healing, and many other ancient shamanic healing rituals around the world, include multi sensory, multi emotional, total cultural, multi medicinal, multi spiritual approaches that mobilize everything that makes up a human being toward one tightly focused goal.

It is this total mental and physical inclusiveness, this ambient richness, that accounts for the frequent success of these ancient disciplines, no matter how "*unscientific*" they undoubtedly are. A modern Western physician, treating AIDS, amounts to sensory deprivation by comparison.

The AIDS patient is unchained from all human connections. Exile is cause for death in many cultures. We are asking a gregarious animal to go off into the desert and cure himself in total solitude. It can't be done. We cannot be healthy alone.

How dare any human being, charged with care for others, coldly ignore the pain in the person in front of him, and think only of blood counts and immune systems! It is truly said that the greatest evil a person can commit is to make another human being into an object.

Does that mean that we have to share our grief, that wisdom must be shared, that healing is shared? You bet it does! The most important act of healing, that the doctor fails to do, is to listen to the patient!

We insist on seeing AIDS as "*their*" problem. Don't we understand how close to us this virus creeps in its silent ugliness? A serpent is prowling the garden of love. Is it the lack of a science of human relations we need to address, or more basically, the issue of our quickness in learning to hate? Blessed are the peace makers, for they shall be crucified?

I discussed this issue the other day with a colleague. At one point he gently leaned toward me and said, "*Gershon, science should concern itself with material progress and leave human nature and social relationships to an unguided moral sense.*" I could only answer that social science will take ages, if ever, to repair the ravages of this world's undirected technology! It seems to me that technology has created as many problems as it has solved.

*Perhaps the most grievous of these failures, in the long run, is the thoughtless development of technical means to cut deaths and increase births, until this world groans under the social and ecological burden of six billion people, soon to be ten billion, and more. All of today's cold medical and legal mechanisms designed to cut certain conditions and groups out of the medical care system are the direct result of this. Calls for legal euthanasia and easy abortion are inevitable.*

What lepers are we stoning today? How well can you be, without your brother's prayers? Who binds the wounds of cruelty? We are told that we were created in God's image. What a vile thing to say of God!

Do we, acting as gods, damn the AIDS patient, or instead place our head upon his pillow and weep? We go about our daily business, politician in control of research dollars, doctor in control of treatment options, mis-managed care organizations, and the bell ringing out "*Leper!*" echoes down the years.

We shut the window, close the drapes, lock the door, turn up the television, and profane all Sabbaths, but if we listen we can still hear the screams in the deepest hour of the night.

Those who worship a God of smoke and flame, give thanks for AIDS, but after homosexuals, drug addicts, and the continent of Africa, the bell will toll for them! Horace said, "*Your own safety is at stake when your neighbor's house is on fire.*"

There is an old story that God called all the angels together before deciding whether to make Man or not. He got a unanimous Yes except for the angel of Truth who voted No. In anger God threw the angel of Truth upon the ground and went ahead. God has learned, since that day, that Truth is the highest angel, and for us, his lack is the highest source of suffering. The battle is within us.

Let our struggle be validated through the most intense personal work a human can do, and if you call it prayer, so be it.

One person in my practice told me, when she was facing a terminally labeled disease, that she used visualization and directed imagery. Why not! Imagine yourself as a warrior with your well honed sword yclept "Kancer Killer", strapped to your side. Mobilize the Tanks and Guns of Light on your behalf. Refuel the Enola Gay and drop The Big A on The Big C. Will you recover? Maybe not. A remote chance is worth seizing, is it not?

Why erode further the plight of the desperate with facts, when what they want is truth? We cannot impose words on wounded people. In spirit and in laughter they may find healing power.

W. H. Auden had the right idea, in the poem Nones, when he wrote:

*Give me a doctor partridge-plump,*
*Short in the leg and broad in the rump,*
*An endomorph with gentle hands*
*Who'll never make absurd demands*
*That I abandon all my vices*
*Nor pull a long face in a crisis,*
*But with a twinkle in his eye*
*Will tell me that I have to die.*

Yes we die. And prayer is not recognized as a cure for AIDS, but in the interim, we can ask if we have mattered? Have we answered or asked the most important questions? There is a texture to healing beyond the surgeon's knife and the internist's injections. Can we at least die, not only with a little dignity, but with confidence?

There are moments when heaven and earth kiss each other, and the veil lifts, opening for our eyes a vision of what is eternal. There are moments when we are ablaze beyond our power.

The nakedness of bare branches and deep roots is the nakedness of the physician before the world. Stripped of his pretensions, he must delve into moral bed rock.

We all eat the dry bread of self affliction, and the bitter root of self delusion. Where is the mitigation? We are clay. Why has not the daughter of my people recovered? Is there no physician there?

1 *Scientific American, March, 1996.*

2 *Discover magazine, June 1996.*

3 *Founder and president, Heimlich Institute, Cincinnati, Ohio, Los Angeles View, 20 October 1995.*

# 15

## The Oath of Hippocrates

There is something extremely beautiful I want to share with you, the ethical heart of this book. This oath is still the ethical heart of Western medicine after 2,300 years. It defines what a physician should be for all time. Hippocrates was the great Greek physician who died in 377 B.C.E. His oath is still sworn by many medical students. It may throw a more bearable light on much of the horror in this book. The tension between what is, what should be, and what could be, has never been more clearly expressed.

*The Oath Of Hippocrates*

> *"I swear by Apollo the physician, by Aesculapius, by Hygeia, Panacea, and all the gods and goddesses, that according to my best ability and judgment, I will keep this oath and stipulation; to reckon him who taught me this art equally dear to me as my parents; to share my substance with him and relieve his necessities if required; to regard his offspring as on the same footing as my own brothers, and to teach them this art if they shall wish to learn it, without fee or stipulation, and that by precept, oral teaching and every other mode of instruction, I will impart a knowledge of the art to my own sons and to those of my teachers, and to disciples bound by a stipulation and oath, according to the law of medicine, but to no others. I will follow that method of treatment, which, according to my ability and judgment, I consider for the benefit of my patients, and abstain from*

*whatever is deleterious and mischievous. I will give no deadly medicine to anyone if asked, nor suggest any such counsel; furthermore, I will not give to a woman an instrument to produce abortion. With purity and with holiness I will pass my life and practice my art. I will not cut a person who is suffering with a stone, but will leave this to be done by practitioners of this work. Into whatever houses I enter I will go into them for the benefit of the sick and will abstain from every voluntary act of mischief and corruption, and further, from the seduction of females or males, bond or free. Whatever in connection with my professional practice, or not in connection with it, I may see or hear in the lives of men which ought not to be spoken abroad, I will not divulge, as reckoning that all such should be kept secret. While I continue to keep this oath inviolate, may it be granted to me to enjoy life and the practice of my art, respected always by all men, but should I trespass and violate this oath, may the reverse be my lot."*

These words still ring like great bells. They are a sad reminder of what we have lost.

Apollo the physician was the patron god of the physicians of ancient Greece, as well as the god of music, poetry, prophecy, and the founding of cities. Apollo's son Aesculapius became more centrally the patron god of physicians. Hygeia, the goddess of health, and Panacea, the divine healer, were daughters of Aesculapius.

In 1948, The Declaration of Geneva was adopted by the General Assembly of the World Medical Association which extends and echoes the old oath. "*I solemnly pledge myself to consecrate my life to the service of humanity. I will give to my teachers the respect and gratitude which is their due; I will practice my profession with conscience and dignity; the health of my patient will be my first consideration; I will respect the secrets which are confided in me; I will maintain by all means in my power the honor and the noble traditions of the medical profession; my colleagues will be my brothers; I will not permit considerations of religion, nationality, race, party politics, or social standing to intervene between my duty and my patient; I will maintain the utmost respect for human life from the time of conception; even under threat, I will not use my medical knowledge contrary to the laws of humanity. I make these promises solemnly, freely, and upon my honor."*

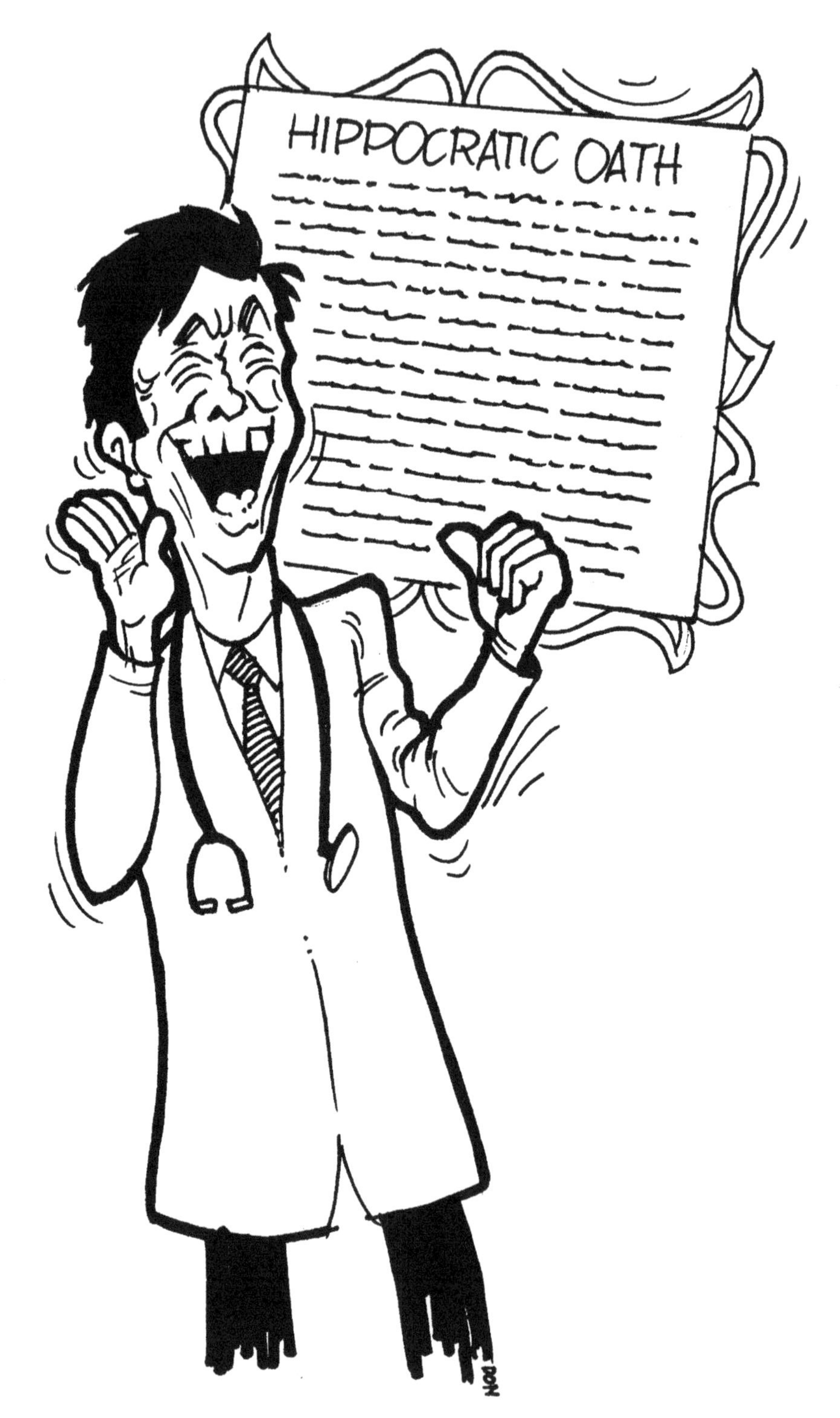
HIPPOCRATIC OATH
DON

# 16

## Doctor Linus Pauling's Last Interview

Dr. Linus Pauling was the only holder in history of two unshared Nobel Prizes, in Chemistry and Peace. He is known to most Americans for his visionary understanding of the role antioxidants would play in our lives, and most famously for his views on the use of vitamin C supplementation.

He was one of the first, as well as one of the last, researchers I interviewed on the air. What follows is the third interview I had with Dr. Pauling in 1993, the last he gave to anyone before his death. As such, it holds some claim to notice by the science of biochemistry and visionaries of alternative and complementary medicine.

Following the usual introduction of my program on KCRW, the interview began:

Good afternoon and welcome to The Health Connection. How does vitamin C play an integral role in your life, is a question listeners continue to write me to ask. To that end, America's vitamin C expert, Dr. Linus Pauling, joins us today as he did 15 years ago, and again 8 years ago, to bring your question up to date, and give us the latest news concerning other vitamins, along with nutrition, as they affect your health. Dr. Pauling has been the recipient of over 40 honorary degrees from universities across America. He is the author of several books including: "*How To Live Longer and Feel Better*;" and "*The Common Cold*."

> Q: Dr. Pauling, each year about 700,000 people develop cancer and most die of it, despite the great amount of money put to cancer research. You present an idea in which you say vitamin C may be used both to prevent cancer and in the treatment of cancer. What is the latest information regarding this relationship?

"High intake of vitamin C, such as I recommend, improves the functioning of the body's natural mechanisms to such an extent as to help to prevent, and help to treat, essentially all diseases. But of course cancer, heart disease, diabetes, the ones that cause the most deaths, are the ones we are especially interested in. I recommend with my friend Dr. Eweren Cameron, who had treated large numbers of patients with advanced cancer by giving them 10 gm (grams) of vitamin C a day, day after day, never stopping. I recommend that every cancer patient take higher doses of vitamin C, in the range of what I myself am taking, which is 18,000 mg (milligrams) a day, in the range of 300 times what the authorities recommend."

> Q: How did you arrive at these dosages?

"Of course the nutrition board recommends only 60 mg a day, which is just enough to keep you from developing scurvy, Yet 25 years ago, I, Dr. Irwin Stone, and Dr. Fred Klemmer all agreed you need far more of this nutrient to be in really good health."

"You know you can't say this about drugs. I think this is what the medical profession doesn't understand. A drug may be valuable in controlling some serious disease and the more you take of it the more chance to control the disease, but all drugs are poisonous, toxic, so that ultimately you would be taking in an amount that would kill you, just because of the toxicity of the drug. Accordingly, a drug used to treat life threatening disease is given in amounts almost to kill by the drug's toxicity. Taking five times the prescribed dose might lead to death. Now the vitamins have essentially no toxicity."

"I doubt any person has ever been killed by an overdose of vitamins, which raises the question, 'How much vitamin C should a person take to prevent disease and be in the best of health, and be of the most value in treating the disease along with any conventional treatment if there is one?' That's a problem I've been working on for 25 years. So Dr. Stone suggested I increase from the RDA of vitamin C which I've been taking for 50 years. He suggested 3 gm a day to prevent colds, especially if you take extra amounts at the first sign of the cold. But after 10 years of more study I went to 6 gm a day (100 times RDA), then to 12 gm a day (200 times RDA), and now I'm up to 18 gm or 300 times RDA for several years, and also taking mega amounts of other vitamins."

"In the case of vitamin C, one fact impressed me very much. I learned about 25 years ago that animals require the same vitamins that humans do. Vitamin C is the exception because most animals don't need any vitamin C in foods because almost all species including fish and insects manufacture their own vitamin C, and the amount they manufacture is, on the basis of body weight, about 200 times RDA. That is to say, animals make, in their own organs, especially the liver, 200 times as much vitamin C as the food and nutrition board recommends for humans. So all living humans are suffering from the disease of hypoascorbemia, not getting enough vitamin C, to be in really good health."

> Q: So, Dr. Pauling, you think nature made a mistake with us, or sometime in our history an event occurred which genetically caused us to cease making it?

"We can ask first, why is it that animals require vitamins while plants manufacture their own? The answer is that when the first animals began eating plants, the plants were making enough vitamin C to keep them healthy, and the other vitamins too, so that the animals were getting by that way. Mutations occurred losing the ability to manufacture all vitamins since they got them in food."

"For vitamin C this didn't happen since the animals require more vitamin C than plants do. Animals use vitamin C to make collagen, the protein that holds our bodies together, including blood vessels and muscles, and skin and bones, teeth and gums, and plants don't need this collagen. They use cellulose as their macromolecular substance, which makes plants strong."

"Animals need much more vitamin C than plants, so they manufacture vitamin C by themselves, except us. A bad accident happened to an early ancestor of human beings, or animals that ultimately became human. This animal was living in the tropical forests where all the fruits and veggies were so high in vitamin C, which animals ate in such large amounts that the animal no longer needed to make vitamin C. The precursor of humans lost the ability to make vitamin C. Since then, we and primates, all similar descendants, have had to find enough vitamin C to keep alive. This was easy, eating tropical fruits. Humans moving out to other regions lost the ability to eat so much of the fruits. Thus humans made pickles and sauerkraut to keep vitamin C available through the winter to keep alive. We still get inadequate amounts to be in good health."

> Q: Is there any danger we can cause ourselves in taking too much vitamin C, and if so, what dangers?

"There is no danger if you mean life threatening, but there is a property of vitamin C that keeps people in ordinary health from taking very large amounts. This is the property of vitamin C to be a laxative. If health is good, higher vitamin C may cause diarrhea. Ill people will find they can take much larger amounts, 60 or 100 gm a day, without getting the laxative effect. Bowel power changes as people are sicker, and as you get well the laxative effect begins to show up again. This is not a danger but probably a good property. It is why people are urged to eat prunes and other fruits containing large amounts of vitamin C."

> Q: Dr. Pauling, if we take vitamin C, what form would you have us take? Is there a better preparation, or is plain ascorbic acid adequate?

"No, there's no special kind. Buy the cheapest. The cheapest is pure crystalline ascorbic acid, or sodium ascorbate. I take the half mixture. I buy these as the cheapest and most convenient way to take large amounts. I take 2 heaping teaspoons a day, dissolved in water, in the morning. I take a vitamin C tablet or two a day. I recommend that every adult take 3 gm a day. Use 2 gm tablet with each meal. It's as convenient."

> Q: In your book, *How to Live Longer and Feel Better*, you write, "Vitamin C controls the misery that plagues the cancer patient." Now, how does it do this? Do you have proof that vitamin C does this, or is there something else involved? Can people who are miserable, but healthy, look forward to the same effect?

"I'm sure there is an effect of vitamin C on mood in some. Of course, if a person has cancer, or other debilitating disease, the body doesn't function well including all the biochemical reactions. This misery, characteristic of debilitating diseases, is a result of the body's inability to function well. High doses of vitamin C allow the body to function well."

> Q: Dr. Pauling, you write that vitamin C slows the aging process. Develop that please.

"I think the main way vitamin C slows aging is in preventing episodes of illness. I have a friend who, years ago, made a study of how much is cut off life expectancy by each episode of illness. Each episode, including a common cold, uses up stores of vitality we have. A person is born with a sum total of vitality. A stressful life uses up this vitality more rapidly. In particular there are illnesses."

> Q: Front page news is that vitamin E may prevent heart attacks and may improve the quality of life. Do you have a comment concerning vitamin E?

"Vitamin E has been known for a long time to protect against heart disease. I wrote a paper on this about 20 years ago, mainly using some biochemical evidence, but also the practical fact that 2 doctors in Canada, Evan and Wilford Schute, treated some 40,000 patients with heart disease by having them take large amounts of vitamin E. I take 800 units daily. That's 50 times the RDA. The Schutes recommended 2,400 units a day. Vitamin E is effective in destroying free molecules which chemically do damage. So are vitamin C and beta carotene antioxidants. Vitamin C is the most effective, E next. I recommend all."

> Q: New studies show extracted plant enzymes might be beneficial to one's health by detoxifying micromolecular debris from nutrition. Do you agree that enzymes such as these will improve life's quality?

"I think that, especially for elders, or those with digestive problems, it is well worth while to use them. Enzymes are large molecules and do not enter the blood system. They work in the intestines, on material consumed, improving digestion. Other enzymes just get digested themselves and never get into the blood stream and do not do what many believe they might."

> Q: Would you care to tell the audience what you think is an appropriate regimen for vitamin supplementation in the 3-1/2 minutes we have left?

"Dr. Hoffer, in Canada, treated 300 patients with advanced cancer, starting with 12 gm of vitamin C, 800 units vitamin E, 30 mg beta carotene, 1,500 mg vitamin B3, and 25 times the RDA of other B vitamins, plus selenium and zinc. Dr. Cameron's book is in its second edition. These results were interesting and better. He got 40 percent of patients with terminal cancer who have now lived for 5 or 10 years after they were judged untreatable."

Q: Dr. Pauling, time makes me quickly ask, in the next minute we have to go, do you think people should be eating sugar?

"I recommend cutting sugar intake to half of ordinary. That's eating perhaps 50 pounds a year instead of 100 pounds. I think meat is valuable but people eat too much of it. Fish is especially valuable. You can find this in '*How To Live Longer and Feel Better.*' The second edition is in the works right now."

Q: May we have the honor of an interview again sometime?

"OK. In the next 8 years I'll be 100 years old. Let's do the next interview then."

Well, if I'm lucky enough, and do what you say, I promise I'll call you back. Thank you for your courage and your vision. Thank you for joining us on the Health Connection. Special thanks to Dorothy Monroe, Dr. Pauling's secretary, for helping arrange this interview.

And that was the last interview ever given by the magic visionary, who died in 1994, at the age of 93. He had not had a cold in 50 years. As he discovered, bringing information to the masses was like a climb up a mountain, or like trying to empty the ocean a spoonful at a time. Yet he did it, while our scientific establishment tried to suppress this wisdom. Miraculously, he would not have it that way.

Stress robs us of our vitality Dr. Pauling said. Indian Chief Gaspesian of the Micmacs said centuries ago that, "*White people have little time for comfort and sweet repose. Anxiety and stress will be the gifts of their progress.*" Anne Schaff said, "*It is not only what the elders say. It is also the way they say it, and what they do with what they say, that gives such wisdom.*"

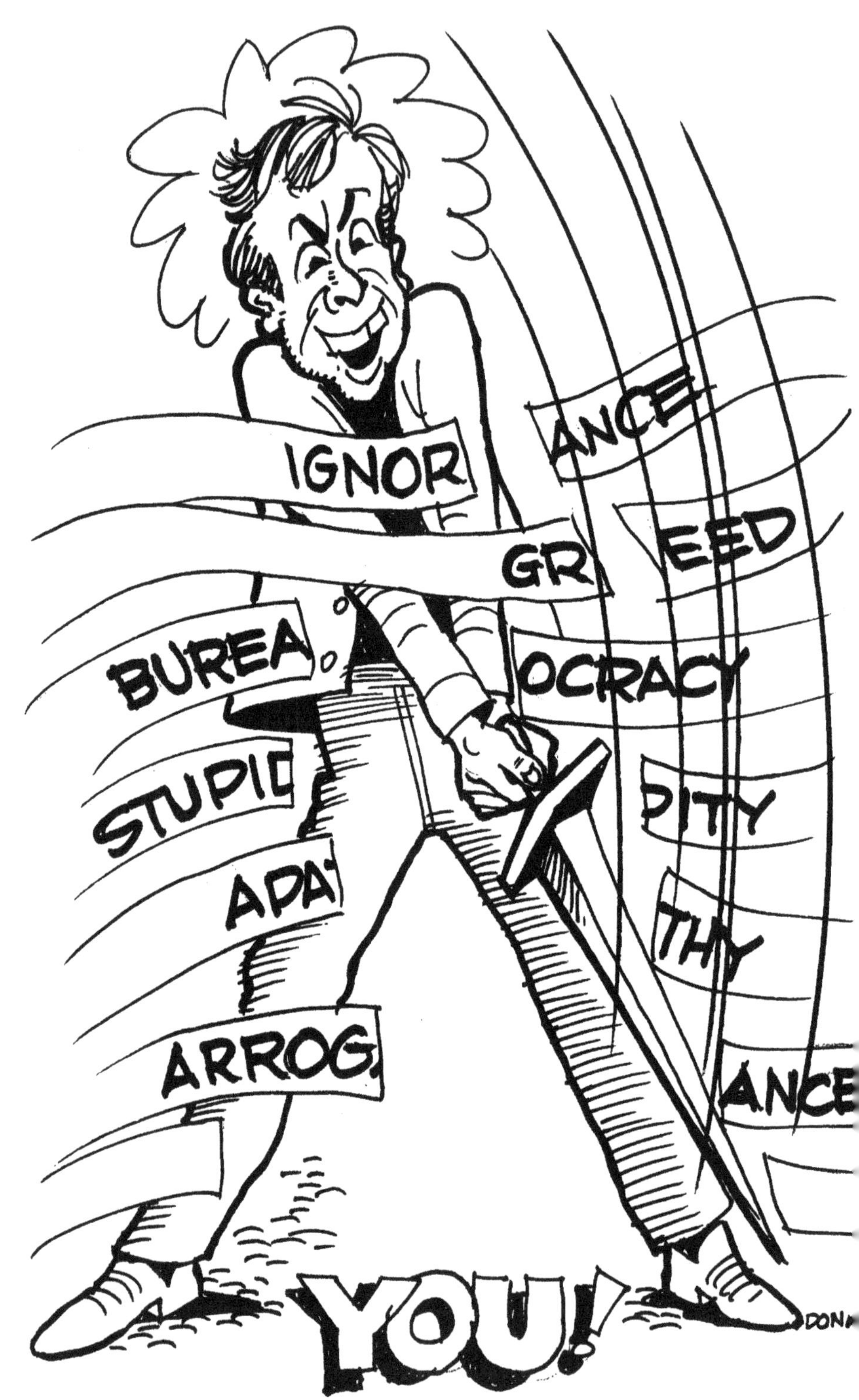

IGNOR
ANCE
GR
EED
BUREA
OCRACY
STUPID
ITY
APA
THY
ARROG
ANCE
YOU!

# 17

## Unicorn's Horn - Eye of Newt

**Part One: The Ballad Of the 20,000 Viberations (sic)**

For a while when I was a child, my parents decided to adopt The Hays Plan, or as my seven year old mind remembers it: "*The Hays Plan of Pocono Haven, New York.*" They may even still be in business. The idea, as I recall, had something to do with keeping the Protein, Carbohydrate, and other food elements in our diet separate. We would eat protein at one meal, other food elements at other meals. What a charming idea. It might even help us lose weight.

I have in front of me as I write an advertisement for a new book advocating the drinking of water, lots of water. The blurb states, "*The author makes a powerful case for the significant role of chronic dehydration in causing numerous health problems, including digestive disorders and ulcers, rheumatoid arthritis, headaches and back pain, elevated blood pressure and cholesterol, diabetes, asthma and allergies, weight problems, and even some emotional disorders.*" I'm drinking a lot more water these days.

I was amazed just this past week at how many ways I am invited to continue my spiritual searchings, and travel triumphant new paths to enlightenment, eternal truth, and health. In the last seven days I have been invited to discover The 2 Great Forces, The 3 Esoteric Energy Centers, The 3 Objects, The 3 Poisons, The 3 Virtuous Seeds, The 3 Qualities, The 3 Principles, The 3 Levels of Inquiry, The 3 Major Realms, The 3 Stages of Transcendence, The 3 Locks, The 3 Qualities of Strength, The 3 Doshas, The 4 Fold Path, The 4 Heavenly Messengers, The 4 Divine Qualities, The 4 Levels of Listening, The 4 Step Guide, The 4 Worlds, The 4 Noble Truths, The 4 Stages of Mastery, The 4th. Way, The 4 Divine Qualities, The 4

Foundations, The 5 Skanddhas, The 5 Wonderful Precepts, The 5 Prostrations, The 5 Remembrances, The 5 Soul Levels, The 5 Faces of Creation, The 5 Difficult Energies, The 5 Yin Organs, The 5 Pillars, The 5 Pranas, The 5 Tones, The 6 Patterns, The 6 Perceptions, The 6 Secret Meditations, The 7 Fruits, The 7 Capital Sins, The 8-Fold Path, The 9 Steps, The 9 Passions, The 9 Virtues, The 12 Steps, The 12 Principles, The 12 Pressure Points, The 32 Secret Paths, The 52 Mental Qualities, The 59 Written Maxims, The 10,000 Joys, and The 10,000 Sorrows.

Also within the past week I have been assured of the lasting efficacy of various applications, belts, straps, and wraps, interventions, lustrations, and penetrations; bars, capsules, cremes, extracts, gels, lotions, lozenges, monitors, oils, powders, shampoos and real poos, sprays, suppositories, tablets, and tonics; and all designed to be variously put on or in the body to the greater glory of my health.

These include various barks from prickly ash, birch, cascara sagrada, cat's claw and catnip, dogwood bark (of course they do), slippery elm, black haw, horehound leaves (ask your grandpa), white oak, the tea tree, willow, witch hazel; various roots including black snake, blood, grape, horse chestnut, horsetail, and marshmallow root (we're more familiar with the fruit, which we roast over picnic fires); the oils of apricot and almond, carrot seed, castor bean, jojoba, and pumpkin seed; various concentrates of raw heart, raw liver (yum!), raw prostate, and raw thymus; astragalus, belladonna, buchu leaves, burdock root, calendula flowers, cayenne, chamomile, red clover, comfrey, corn silk, cubeb (ask your grandpa again), yellow dock (not related to updock), echinacea, feverfew, ginger, goldenseal, lemon grass and shavegrass, nettle, peach leaves, passion flowers, golden rod, sarsaparilla, and watermelon seed; mutton tallow (sheep fat), charcoal, creosote, pine tar, silicon, powdered pearls and powdered metallic silver. After all that I feel a little dizzy, and badly in need of a tonic!

And to make my life complete, this week I have been given the opportunity to find the true ancient way (nutritionally speaking) from many ancient Chinese remedies, with ancient Latin names, including various semens from semen cassiae toreae, semen litchi, semen plartaginis, semen arneniacae, semen cuscutae, and semen sesami (quaint names), dong quai (fittingly) or in Latin radix angelicae sinensis - very trendy these days; various other radixes such as radix bupleuri, radix gentianae, radix ginseng (panax ginseng), radix glycyrrizae, radix morindae, radix polygoni multiflori, radix rehmanniae, radix saussureae, radix scrophularia (ugh!), radix scutellariae, radix salviae multiorhizae, radix sileris, and radix trichosanthis; also rehmanniae glutnosa, plus various rhizomas including rhizoma acori graminei, rhizoma atractylodes curcumae, rhizoma batatis, and rhizoma sparganii; also bulbus fritillariae roylei, fructus bardebae, amoni cardamomi, ramulus cinnamonum; some flosses such as flos cathami, flos chrysanthemi, and flos magnoliae; cortex moutan radicis, gynostemma, codonopsis; poria, shiitake, and tea funguses; jiaogulan, byplerum, herba lamnae and herba artemisiae capillaris, meliae toosendan, and blue cohosh (caulophylum thalictroides), as well as other flowers (flos), fruit (fructus), barks (cortex), bulbs (bulbus), rhizomes (sort of a root), and roots (radix). I'll bet that everything above is the Latin name of everything in the previous paragraph. Do you take these remedies without thinking? I sure don't! Problems may lie in wait.

In the interest of health these remedies promise to absorb, arrest, clarify, clean, cure, favor, flush, knit, ream, rejoin, renew, resorb, reverse, tone up, and unify; all the arteries, bones, cartilages, discs, joints, ligaments, muscles, nerves, organs, tendons, tissues, veins; of the body which have been abraded, boiled, broken, bruised, burned, compressed, contused, cut, dislocated, fractured, gangrened, infected, inflamed, lacerated, narrowed, punctured, ruptured, sprained, strained, separated, suppurated, swollen, torn, tumored, wenned, and wrenched. As Jean Kerr said, "*I'm tired of all this nonsense about beauty being only skin deep. That's deep enough. What do you want - an adorable pancreas?*"

It is my expectation that when I have mastered all these joys and sorrows I will disappear in two clearly separated puffs of protein and carbohydrate fog to be translated directly to the 50 Yard Line at Pocono Haven, New York, with an urgent desire to urinate. I don't suppose it's necessary to spell out the moral of all this?

**The concept of the "*general purpose tonic*" needs to be retired from use.** So far as I know, there is no medication which functions to tone up the body in a general sense, no product which can be taken without regard to any complaint, nothing you can put in your mouth that cannot be abused, even water. You have to use herbs safely and that means don't overdo them and don't take them when you're pregnant! Take your mind and heart along!

**Part Two: Chinese Black Balls**

Onward. Chinese Black Balls (Yikes!), are supposed to be an ancient and glorious remedy proved by "*thousands of years of peasant use*," right? Well, actually, no! We are told the story of one 71 year old user of Chinese Black Balls who developed a bleeding ulcer because she was exceeding the recommended dose of a well known anti inflammatory drug called mefensamic acid which had somehow crept into her ancient remedy.

We hear of woman number two who also took Chinese Black Balls. In the hospital emergency room it turned out that her kind of Black Balls contained 7 mg. of Valium, much too much for someone unused to the drug. Valium is not an ancient Chinese remedy either. Other Black Balls, sold over a period of 20 years, have been found to contain Librium, steroids such as prednisone, muscle relaxants, and diuretics, not to mention contaminants like lead.

Suffering people looking for any relief they can get should not adopt a "What have I got to lose?" attitude. The answer could be, "*Your life!*"

Don't fill a doctor's prescription and assume the ancient remedy you are now taking doesn't already contain a large dose of the same drug. Talk to your doctor and he will talk to you. If your doctor knows nothing about herbs, try talking to a pharmacist who also sells herbs. As I have said before, too often we upset delicate and complex balances and then must deal with the results. Restraint is needed.

People will never think twice about an herb, who might understand the disaster of taking some patented drug without thought. Any chemical which can heal us can hurt us! Just because you call it herbal doesn't mean it can't be abused.

Most people are using an herb called coffee. Large amounts of coffee are toxic. You can get headaches, get nervous, go crazy, be unable to sleep, get ringing in the ears, become dizzy, get cardiac arhythmias. There is no right amount with some natural products. After all, opium is "*natural*," and cocaine is "*organic*" I suppose.

Some other serious herbs that I think people should stay away from, which I have heard being recommended by some herbalists, include water hemlock, dong quai, and belladonna. Another herb commonly used for allergies and colds, goldenseal, is also something to be worried about.

There are some herbs from India which leave residues of arsenic or lead or other heavy metals in the body. Other herbs that can cause serious harm, and should not be used, are Chaparral, responsible for at least 6 cases of acute nonviral hepatitis; Comfrey, linked to at least 7 cases of obstructed blood flow from the liver, with potential cirrhosis (scarring), one person died; Ephedra (ma huang, epitonin, Mormon Tea, less than a capsule can cause harm - see below); and Yohimbe, really big at this writing although evidence for its efficacy is "*sparse and inconclusive*," and overdoses can cause weakness and nervous stimulation followed by paralysis, stomach disorders, and ultimately even death. Most users get away with it, but it's taking too great a chance.

Certain labelling and purity guidelines won't go into effect for several years. Products can go to market with no testing for efficacy. The manufacturers do not have to prove that herbal products are safe. Supplements do not have to be manufactured according to any standards, even the basics of quality control are not yet enforced. Label claims might not have much evidence behind them. And FDA approval is not needed. This last may not be all that bad, but we should be extremely careful.

The world is dangerous, our pharmaceutical companies are dangerous, even the natural time tested remedies can be dangerous. Life is dangerous. If we bring our mind and our heart along, then we can be dangerous too and we may not have to bring Big Brother along, to protect us from ourselves!

Before you take one of these ancient remedies, at least you should know the product's scientific name and plant parts used, the name and address of the manufacturer, batch and lot number, and dates of manufacture and expiration.

I talked to Rolling Thunder, medical man and legal advisor for the Western Shoshone nation, many years ago, who was pleased to tell me that he thought he had just rediscovered a medicine, combining physical and mystical qualities, long thought to be lost forever to the Shoshone. He had just tried it. The Indian medical man earns our respect the hard way.

The problem with folklore is that we can't be guaranteed, or even know, the proper dosage. Someone has to try it. The final product may not be pure, or may have possible contamination by preservative and insecticidal sprays. Some of the active ingredients have not yet been identified. Herbalism is still disorganized and not fully scientific. Probably your best, and only, defense in regard to herbals is a highly respected company label.

On the other hand, herbalists have always known something modern science is only just beginning to recognize; synergy, or the multiplication of a drug's action when all the parts of a plant are used or when components of several plants are put together, which sometimes reveals new uses or powers, and an unexpected effectiveness.

Please note that no one can claim any of the herbal remedies are a "*cure*" for anything. What we're talking about is an active positive move in diet toward certain herbs and nutrients which are expected to help the body remain healthy. Most medical doctors wouldn't give a second thought to them, as yet. They would not tell you, as I will, that my list of supplements would include green tea rather than any other kind, garlic, ginger, and of course astragalus which is now available, and maitake which is becoming available.

**Part Three: MA HUANG - Ephedrin**

BEWARE! So-called "*designer drugs*," notably "*Herbal Ecstacy* (sic)," are available over-the-counter, and mail order, as legal highs, due mainly to the ingredient Ma Huang (epitonin, Mormon Tea), an "*all natural*" Chinese herb which contains ephedrin and which possesses amphetamine-like properties. Some of the products also contain caffeine. Similar products are popular as performance enhancers, and weight control aids, for athletes and body builders.

Like the amphetamines, the ephedrines are classified as nervous system stimulants, often causing jitters, anxiety, and headaches. Less than the amount contained in one capsule can cause harm. It can raise blood pressure, cause heart palpitations, nerve damage and muscle injury, psychosis, stroke, and memory loss. Deaths have occurred! Medical authorities worry that users are risking serious health problems including heart attack. People with heart and thyroid conditions, high blood pressure, and those taking anti depressants are at risk. So are those sensitive to it, or overdosing. The FDA says it has received more than 300 reports of adverse effects including a dozen deaths involving persons who consumed ephedrin alkaloids.

Several states have started to restrict their sale. The Ohio State Pharmacy Board for instance is only allowing ephedrin products to be sold prescriptively. Better stay away.

**Part Four: Stevia**

What about artificial sweeteners? Saccharine has been sold commercially since 1900, predating the FDA. The FDA attempted to ban it in 1977 but Congress responded to public outcry and now mandates a warning about possible cancer causing properties instead.

Aspartame was approved by the FDA for widespread us in 1983. It has shown side effects occasionally such as headaches, dizziness, mood changes, numbness, nausea and vomiting, muscle cramps and spasms, abdominal pain, vision problems, skin lesions, memory loss, and seizures. Individuals with PKU, approximately one in every 14,000 people, should not use it. About 75 percent of all non-drug complaints to the FDA are about aspartame.

A third sweetener, acesulfame potassium, was licensed in 1988 for limited uses.

The latest artificial sweetener, the fourth to be approved by the FDA, is "sucralose" which is 600 times sweeter than sugar. No warning about potential health problems will have to be posted with the product, based on a review by the FDA of more than 110 animal and human studies, although one high dosage test on animals showed shrinkage of the thymus gland, part of the body's immune system. Sucralose is a chemical variant of ordinary sugar, i.e. sucrose.

Refined sugar in moderation is still probably better for you than all those sugar substitutes. I worry about sugar substitutes possibly inducing brain disorders, from headaches to mood and emotional changes. They have also been suggested as possible cancer inducers or birth defect related. Artificial sugar substitutes seem to have caused one of my patients a severe colitis.

Stevia is an economical natural sweetener used for generations in Paraguay. It is in major use in Japan. One teaspoon of dried ground stevia leaves is said to be as sweet as a cup of sugar. It may be helpful to people who are diabetic, prone to yeast infections, or trying to lose a few pounds. It can likely help fight tooth decay as well. It is available widely in vitamin stores but is not well known. No one has a patent on it which may explain the lack of advertising, When refined it has no appreciable flavor of its own. Cooking does not destroy its sweetness. I know of no important side effects.

**Part Five: Saw Palmetto**

Saw palmetto is used regularly in Europe for benign prostate hypertrophy (BPH - an enlarged prostate) at a cost of 35 cents a day, far less than the accepted pharmaceuticals, which cost up to two dollars a day, and can have troubling side effects.

I see in the papers that the saw palmetto berry had Florida in a frenzy a couple of years ago. For some reason the flowers dropped off too early and the prices being paid for the berries went from 10 cents a pound to as high as $3.50 a pound for awhile. The center of the trade is Immokalee, in the Everglades, near the Seminole Indian reservation, Pickups and family vans searching for berries were reported to be breaking down fences onto private land, and letting the cows out onto the highways.

Stories called the saw palmetto (Serenoa repens) a "*reputed aphrodisiac*," and got a few other things wrong, but they did point out that all through the southeastern U.S. the saw palmetto is considered a nuisance by the farmers and ranchers, about on a par with the kudzu vine, which you'll note is also showing up in herb remedies these days. How long before the imported water lily choking so many ponds and streams in the southeast, as well as the imported western tumbleweed, are "*rumored*" to be aphrodisiacs?

Everything is connected to everything else, and health is no longer a personal decision. Men in Europe and the United States are worried about their enlarged prostates, and Florida goes crazy.

Just consider some of the aspects of this story. The Seminole Indians, for instance. Do you think they like this latest mass invasion of the White Man onto their reservation? The commercial growers hire migrants to pick the berries. Doesn't that push a few political buttons? What about those broken fences? It sure doesn't make the insurance companies happy when a cow and a car meet at 65 MPH on a Florida highway. The wild boars and the rattlesnakes also seem to be getting a little nervous out there in the bush.

And when you look at this story carefully, don't you see parallels with the old Chinese gentleman who "*needs*" powdered rhinoceros horn to assuage the regrets of an impotent old age? It's probably a good thing that Viagra is not a natural product.

The rhinoceros will soon be extinct, and who will note the passing of one more of The Million Things, except perhaps for God? Health is becoming the most pressing, all inclusive, and political, issue of all!

Abraham J. Heschel said, "*Faith is not a feature of Man's mentality. It is not self effacement of curiosity, asceticism of reason, or some psychic quality that has bearing on man alone. The essence of faith is not disclosed in the way we utter it, but in the soul's being in accord with that which is really relevant, in our being carried away by the tide of universal thoughts, rising beyond the desolate ken of Man's despair.*"

**Part Six: Taxol**

Our teeming billions won't wipe out the saw palmetto, but they were well on the way to wiping out the pacific yew tree a few years ago, searching for a remedy for cancer in its bark. Taxol, the active ingredient in the yew, was found in the tree's needles just in time. Cutting of the tree was halted in 1993. A 100 year old tree provided only a gram of the compound, about half the amount needed for a single treatment. Next year will it be pup fish gristle? Or maybe spotted owl spots?

*"They can arrange for loggers to find more meaningful work, but by god sir! - that's my prostate you're discussing!"*

Considered one of the most promising treatments for breast and ovarian cancer, and possibly effective against lung cancer and melanoma, Taxol may have some troubling side effects, especially in the stock market. An entire group of "*taxoids*" are now being studied. There is more on cancer in Chapters six and thirteen.

I'm sure you realize that I have not attempted to deal thoroughly with the subject of herbal remedies here. There are hundreds available, with varying amounts of information at hand. The entire field of medicine is changing too rapidly to keep entirely up to date.

Racing ahead of the power saws of the lumbermen are a few entrepreneurs of medicine. They are looking for new natural remedies used by the tribal medical men in the remaining natural forests of the world. Both the forests and the medical men have an ever shorter life span, so there is some urgency to the search.

It has taken us only three generations to remove the earth's top soil and forests. The genetic treasures of the ages, the creations of God, are under the plow and the power saw. All future generations are being impoverished.

After all, approximately 25 percent of the drugs we already use are derived from plants. And less than 1 percent of natural plant sources have been studied by the medical drug companies. Maybe only 1 in 10,000 plants can be economically turned into a prescription drug but that's still a lot of money to the drug companies in the developed world. The benefits to us would be immense.

The Indian medical men don't get anything out of it of course. Too bad. They can always meditate while sitting on one of the tree stumps, or move to the slums of Rio or Bogota and get drunk.

Lord, I thank thee for this world of color, space, movement, and intent. I thank thee for The Million Things. Amen.

- *Chinese Medicine information: Director of UCLA Center of East-West Medicine, 1(310) 794-6644.*

- *The American Association of Naturopathic Physicians can give you information about herbs. The number is (206) 323-7610.*

- *The Food and Drug Administration will give you the official view of herbs at (800) 332-1088.*

- *I highly recommend 2 books by Varro Tyler. The first is "The New Honest Herbal: A Sensible Guide to the Use of Herbs and Related Remedies", 3rd. ed., organized by herb, 1993, published by Pharmaceutical Products Press.*

- *The second is "Herbs of Choice: The Therapeutic Use of Phytomedicinals", organized by disease, 1994, V.E. Tyler, Pharmaceutical Products Press.*

- *"Phytotherapy: A Practical Handbook of Herbal Medicine for the Practitioner", 1989, Dr. Demargaux, Surrey Press.*

- *"German Commission E Monographs on Medicinal Plants for Human Use", 1997, The American Botanical Council, 327 herbal remedies. The German herbal bible.*

- *"The Complete Herbal", by Dr. B. C. Harris, 1972, published by Barre.*

- *"Herbal Medicine", 1988, R.F. Weiss, Medicina Biologica*
- *The Honest Herbal: A Sensible Guide to the Use of Herbe and Related Remedies". 1993, V.E, Tyler, Pharmaceutical Products Press.*
- *"The Scientific Validation of Herbal Medicine", by Dr. Mowrey, 1986, published by New Canaan.*
- *"Clinical Homeopathic Materia", vol. 1, by Dr. Tetau, 1986, Paris.*
- *"Planetary Herbology" by Dr. Tierra, 1988, published in Santa Fe.*
- *"The Vitamin and Herb Guide", 1992, by Global Health, Ltd.*
- *"Handbook of Medicinal Herbs", 1987, J.A. Duke, CRC Press.*

*Of varying usefulness may be the following net addresses. Beware of typos.*

*1.) netvillage.com/ 2.) herbalgram.org 3.) pitt.edu/~cbw/atlm.html 4.) ars-grin.gov/ngrlsb 5.) healthy.net/*

*Directory of Databases (summary of U.S., Europe, and Asia):*

*http://CPMCNET.columbia.edu/dept/rosenthal/databases/AM_databases.html*

*U.S. Department of Agriculture, Agriculture Genome Information System (taxonomy and worldwide use of herbs):*
*http://probe.nalusda.gov*

# 18

## Never, Never, Never, Never Give Up!

You've probably seen a marvelous and often reprinted cartoon. It shows a big billed bird swallowing a frog. Even as the frog's head begins going down the bird's throat, the frog has his fingers chokingly tight around the bird's neck. The caption sometimes says: "*Never, never, never, never give up!*" Most of us have not yet made that kind of commitment, but all of us are capable of it. Without tenacity, you and I will probably be defeated, no matter what our creativity, our intelligence, or our sensitivity.

In Midrash Tanhuma, Yitro 8, it is written, "*There is no affliction discernible, for which there does not exist a cure; If you seek that misfortune befall not your body, engage in all the acts of study, love, life, and joy, and find even in these there is therapy for the entire body.*"

In spite of all the armaments of medicine, it's your focus, your fear, your anger, your paralysis, the amount of your determination, your view of what can or cannot be accomplished, that must be faced if you are to be healed.

A doctor must understand pain and confusion, the price of fear and anger and insecurity. This is not the kind of thing you ask of the person who sneers at you as you buy stamps at the post office. If we are interested in health giving, we cannot become bureaucrats.

One heretical doctor believes that the benefits of the internet are going to far outweigh the drawbacks. He believes that if people have access to the same information doctors use, they can challenge doctor's orders, take more active control of their own treatment, even find important resources their doctors might have missed.

That opinion will probably send chills of horror up the backs of a lot of doctors, but it seems to me that he's right. **The average intelligent layman is smart enough and motivated enough to**

**become a real expert in her own condition, and if she does so, she should be treated as such.**

I could multiply this little lesson indefinitely. Isn't it clear that everyone needs more information? It is also clear that our well being has a whole lot to do with politics. Political Action Committees (PACs) are not good for our health. We are all smart enough to know our best interests when we see them - if we have access to information. I have a certain amount of optimism these days because so many people, just like you, are beginning to understand what I am getting at here.

**Or have you found this chapter rough going? Does it seem as though I am asking you to do something I have no right to ask of you? Do my invitations seem strange to you? Has freedom begun to sound subversive? And health Un-American?**

The more information you get, the better, but be careful. You might not believe everything that great-aunt Pearl tells you about her chilblains, her ague, or her vapours, but some total stranger can tell you the same thing with shining chromium words on the http://www.dot.edu and you're ready to try it. Can brain fever be far away?

We are not "*the masses.*" We are not "*rabble.*" We are not "*riffraff.*" We are not "*peasants.*" We are not "*those elements.*" Unfortunately we are not "*citizens*" either. We will not be citizens until we somehow manage to pry open the channels of information once again, until we become that "*informed citizenry*" mentioned in our founding documents. It reminds me of an old political sardonicism: "*If the people don't cooperate, we'll just have to abolish them, and appoint a new one.*"

We need all the information we can get. Beginning in the 1920's science fiction readers started publishing their own amateur fan magazines to discuss the writing they loved. These "*zines*" as they were called, have since spread to hundreds of different fields of interest on and off the internet. They are opinionated, vital, full of dubious information (all of which needs to be checked), and often outrageous, a fine late flowering of freedom of the press and, like the old Soviet "*samizdat*," often the only way to disseminate their publisher's opinion, with more traditional publishing sources no longer available to ordinary Americans.

Health and nutrition zines are no exception to this trend, with titles such as "*Take Back Your Life: Wimmin's* (sic) *Guide to Alternative Health,*" "*The Gentle Survivalist: Orion Report,*" "*The Wild Foods Forum,*" and "*The Civil Abolitionist.*" You'll have to keep your eyes open for names and addresses if you are interested. So far as I know, these zines have not yet developed the equivalent of the science fiction field's Amateur Press Association (APA), although I do have one address for a central source for information which may remain accurate temporarily. Prepare to be annoyed.

*Factsheet Five* is a zine about zines with reviews of over 1000 zines of all kinds, records, books, and other marginalia in every issue. The address is R. Seth Friedman, FACTSHEET FIVE, P.O.Box 170099, San Francisco, CA 94117-0099. Send $5.00 for each issue. <f5seth@sirius.com>

Those titles above are likely to be obsolete by the time this book sees print, everything changes so fast. These are manifestations of basic human freedom, rising up from the wellsprings. Remember that even the old USSR never managed to close down their samizdat (zines).

Our rulers seldom remember that in a democracy, power flows from below, and we are the person who needs information the most. We cannot be healthy alone. If something is going wrong, it's because *we* don't have enough information! All information about anything (Yes!) should be available to anyone who wants it, or believes he or she has a use for it. Congress may have to be taught, once again, Jefferson's cold lesson about liberty.

Malcolm Little was a peaceful, smart, and tender little boy. He wrote, "*One thing in particular that I remember made me feel grateful toward my mother was that one day I went and asked her for my own garden, and she did let me have my own little plot. I loved it and took care of it well. I loved especially to grow peas. I was proud when we had them on our table. I would pull out the grass in my garden by hand when the first little blades came up. I would patrol the rows on my hands and knees for any worms and bugs, and I would kill and bury them. And sometimes when I had everything straight and clean for my things to grow, I would lie down on my back between two rows, and I would gaze up into the blue sky at the clouds moving and think all kinds of things.*" Malcolm was not allowed to be healthy alone. What did we do to our brother to turn Malcolm Little into Malcolm X? We create our own judges and arrange our own justice do we not?

There are always lines to divide us. We must learn how to cross the lines. My neighbor's "*unreasoning anger*," is not good for my health, nor is mine good for his!

Most of us cherish our gang, our class, our families, our race, and dislike those others over there. Where? Almost anywhere! It's not fair! What isn't? Almost everything! Of course we are tense all the time.

We can't understand their language. We can't understand their religion. We can't understand their actions and their opinions. We can't understand children at all, even our own. We are exiles in our own world, and we can't go out and murder someone anymore! We're terribly alone and afraid!

In spite of it all, practically everyone tries to be fair. Almost everyone tries to give the other person the benefit of the doubt. Practically everyone keeps their opinions to themselves and hopes for the best.

**No one is paying us the credit due us for our almost constant bravery in the face of provocation that would have led to mass murder in any past age. We are all incredibly and almost constantly marvelous, and no one dares say it to us.**

I'm not talking just to my peers, and my family, and my professional cohorts, even to my readers, although they deserve this credit too. I am talking, for instance, of America's blacks who, despite daily reminders that they are still considered inferior, do not often break down into insanity and riot. Here, in the belly of the beast, they laugh and think and create! What marvelous humanity, vitality and beauty!

I am talking of America's Latinos, trying to support families, often made large by their ethnicity, unable to understand the surrounding Anglo culture, their religion of lessening comfort to them, and yet who still work hard, raise and love their families, and laugh more than they have a right to. These people are incredible.

I am also talking of American families of many oriental cultures and many languages, trying to keep their ancient traditions of family and study alive where there is no outside support. Their beauty and courage is legendary!

I celebrate the cultural splendor of the Jews in America. What would our world be without them - Freud, all the great musicians and writers, Einstein, thought, humor and the joys of Yinglish? The rest of us will always desperately need their quiet reminders that the Cossacks still ride!

And most of all, I am talking to those who should be most at home here, who are still being made unwelcome in their own land, their languages and cultures still being taken from them, the American Indian. Miraculously some of them still remember how to live on this great sweet Turtle Island, our Mother, the Earth. We still repeat (Oh yes we do!) the old saying, "*The only good Indian is a dead Indian,*" and make alcoholism easy for them everywhere. After hundreds of years they still dream and sing and feel at home!

I am proud of Los Angeles, where I live. Not for the reasons put forth, ad nauseam, by the Chamber of Commerce of course, but because it is the second largest city of some 40 countries around the world. There are no minorities in L.A. because there is no longer a majority, white or any other color. Over 100 languages are spoken in the City of the Angels, and the food and music, the dance and art, the laughter and richness of culture of the marvelous people who create this rainbow, are to be cherished by everyone, in spite of the myopia of City Hall and the police. America is still rich in its cultural diversity, still unique in the world.

America was never one tribe, America was never all white, America was never all Protestant, and if we would only remember it, America has always been an idea, an idea of Freedom for all, never a group of WASPS trying to turn our country into a corner of Olde

Englande or Olde Germanye. Ignoring that fact is an invitation to ill health and hate.

Are we brave enough to sing? Our battle is for health! Singing makes our thinking active, not reflexive. It gets our passions flowing. We rise. All of our flags fly. We astound the nurses. Cry if we must; then sing! If we cannot sing, perhaps we can chant. Never give up.

Laughter is a vital part of life. The ability to look in the mirror of life and see the humor, the ridiculous nature of our ambitions, our pretenses and masks, the comedy of our storm and fury, is critical to our survival. We grow up on the day we first laugh at ourselves.

At the end of our century of degradation and genocide and war, our nerve is shattered. What is left of our arts celebrate closure and chaos. We are fouling our nest. Generations of barbarians burn our cities. Yet I cannot help but feel that a vast and shining surprise can await us. Somehow I feel, amidst the rubble, that we are almost ready to fly!

Out of the night comes hope! Don't you feel it? Don't you sense, beyond rational expectation, a breath of air? A door has opened somewhere in the darkness!

Let us imagine how it might be! Can't you hear the bells? Imagine that we have all regained our hope. Open the door and let the joyous laughing crowd in.

Yes, there is grief. Don't luxuriate in it, or you lose your healing motive. We start in the abyss and step by step, never giving up, we rebuild, grabbing onto each day and each other, filling the void with the reality of love, and through our tears, begin to feel joyous health return. Reckon with the bitter roots and the dry bones, but know that there may be flowers, and perhaps atonement (at-one-ment!). Mindfulness is recommended by the highest authority.

Surround yourself with supportive people. We can't find sanity and health alone. We can't deal with our pain alone. The old nuclear family with 2.7 children and a dog and cat is gone forever, but there is more than one way to share love.

So many of us still believe that fate is written in stone by the gods, or we think Fortuna still roles her dice, but neither is true. We create our own future out of what we are now choosing. If we want health in the future, we must be healthy in this moment. Dogmatic certainty plants dragons, not flowers, and reaps the whirlwind! We are in danger of being destroyed by our certainty. Science and a few religions agree that everything is change. Every change in our mind flowers into new universes.

I know this sounds like "*guru-speak*" but try to understand it. Each of us should be aware that our deepest experiences can be full of mind and light. I am talking of the most difficult work any of us can do - but it can be done. We can actualize ourselves!

The Dalai Lama described a classic meditation, "*I would hope that you could learn to sit as if you were a mountain, because a mountain is majestic and it is unshakable. It is in itself at ease with the universe as well as with itself. It is relaxed, and no matter the forces that strike upon it, no matter how dark the clouds that swirl around it, it is steadfast and unshakable. Sit like a mountain, and allow your minds to soar.*"

What I'm asking of us all is a celebration of personal disarmament. Let our guns fall silent. I ask you to reach with me into the rainbow, in the spray and wrack of life's journey, as we search for fertility, for meaning, and resolution.

The world tries to tear us one from another, if not by death, then with age, manipulations of ignorance and inattention, religious conflict rooted in the past, meaningless patter of status and pecking order, subtleties of education and degree and certificate that matter not at all down here where we live together on this green earth. Buddhism teaches that one of the root causes of most suffering is our ignorance.

Has there ever been any moment when it was more important for people to realize the nature of the enormous power and the untapped resources within themselves, and how to use them for themselves and for the sake of their world, than right now?

Dear friends, we are not impostors. We are the authors! We can't forget our lines because we make up our own lines in this play as we go along, and we deserve to succeed. Yes success is frightening, but we have our own life to live, in our own country, as well as we can learn how.

The dull realities and inertias of power hide all those hidden people on our block who have thought deeply. They hide so much information, which is so easily available just off the media beaten track. We are lost in a fog, but overhead the sun is shining. There are a lot of caring and courageous people out there. and we're all in this together.

What is holding us back, and perpetuating the "*same old same old*" until we are all going crazy, is the very thing that has accompanied every decline in human history: inertia, the "*silent majority,*" the needs of power ("*Apres moi le deluge!*"). We tell ourselves that the grim old men will never give in, will never move, that no compromise is possible. This is not true. We must never give up. The secret is that they are terrified of us!

We can choose to make miracles happen. We can stop blaming our mother, the boss, city hall, Congress, or the next tin pot would-be dictator preaching at us in the TV wilderness. We see the destruction so close ahead, but seldom notice the healing and happiness that is also just an act of universal kindness away.

We must begin - and we must never, never, never, never give up. Our lives can have dignity once again. It may be that we can choose to continue the creation of the world.

Health, in its broadest sense, is indistinguishable from citizenship and civilization, and ultimately is a measure of our freedom. Whether you know it or not, your doctor is inviting you to be free.

and Never -

Never -

Never -

Give up!

# 19

## Have You Had Enough?

We have been down some strange roads in this book. I hope it has become clear that you and I are far more than any one view of us can take in. I know that we are meat, and yet we are holy too, aren't we? We are machines and we are spirit. Everything we do is part of everything we are, and the world resonates within all of us.

I use the word "*humanism*" proudly. I am aware of the uses ignorance has made of the word. By humanism I mean the affirmation of human life as central to our meaning and our spirit. We are interested in life here on earth, and care to understand it, and make it better. Humanism is life and joy for every one of us. By humanism I mean the affirmation of ourselves.

So, if we are ill, let us be impassioned in our affirmation. It may take courage but it opens us to healing. It opens us to the good foods, the good people, the games and play and exercise of life. Understanding, awakening, love, they are the same. Join them and we cure the world. Humanism includes our love of nature, of the good in our fellow humans, of our relationship to God. It opens us to wholeness.

We must cultivate the preciousness of every individual person and human dignity, within a culture that must learn to celebrate these values. We must give up suppressive intolerance. We must respect intimacy and honest interpersonal relationships. I say one last time, we cannot be healthy alone. A society that is civilized need not worry about guns in the streets, or love with the improper stranger.

People everywhere are ready for sanity. To deny this, as forces throughout the world wish to do today, distorts the whole of life. We are all wounded, some of us mortally.

We are responsible for our behavior. It is as psychologically naive to acquit the killer because of his prior poverty, as it is to acquit the

CEO because of her lust for profit. The lawyer who damns justice, is responsible for his manipulation of it. Each of us is responsible for our place in the world.

In this light, I feel that it is important to talk a bit more about my reasons for quitting the practice of medicine. Personal tragedy played a role of course, but I would no longer be practicing medicine even if my life had not changed otherwise. As with all independent and private physicians today, I was being ground between the jaws of increasing costs, malpractice insurance, government regulations and the hired help needed to administer the new paper work needed to keep me out of jail. I had only two choices, to sign on at an HMO or equivalent, or retire. There is a tornado whirling its destructive energy throughout the entire health care profession. Its chaos has not been limited to professionals however. You are being tossed into the maelstrom.

Bland acceptance, going along, fitting in, seem to be expected among professionals in medicine. I don't know what course others may take, but I cannot go quietly. No wonder I betray my fury here and there.

Never doubt that physicians are morally and legally expected to render the best, most complete and competent service to sick people. Now they are trying to do so while handcuffed and bound by nonprofessional powers and entities such as mis-managed care HMOs, and government actions, all of which expand their profit agenda by denying services, medicines, and procedures.

It was this upheaval from which I was forced to resign. My medical vision enhances energetic imaginative care. It honors you. I believe in words of healing, of cure, hope, faith, and the limitless possibilities and boundaries in seeking wholesome health. In these times of megabytes of progress in the material, technical world it offends the core morality of my soul when I am told that the treatment of a person of any age is just too expensive and must be denied.

Medicine is no longer the appropriate label for what is really "*illness servicing*." The physician is no longer the hand holding and caring doctor, but has turned into a "*provider*." Providers do not have to care. They don't even have to be courteous.

This is venture capital at work at its moral worst. Your health care is not a physician's interest any more. It is a Wall Street issue. The social cost is immense. You are now part of the health industry. You perceive yourself as a customer paying a premium to insure your future, but too often you are kidding yourself.

Whether you live or die from cancer now depends as much as on when someone decides it's finally time to check you, as how much will be allotted dollar wise for treatment. Your doctor's "*art*" is removed.

If you are ill, old, poor, disabled, anything but absolutely healthy, or absolutely wealthy, you are a serious risk for health insurers and government cash flow. You may not be aware of it but in many of these categories there are accountants explaining how it is you aren't worth the cost. You diminish profit, and are then denied adequate care.

This is a revolution in which the corporation evolves, no matter how mangled and compromised the health care becomes. **NO!** I could not remain morally involved as a doctor, forced to compromise the very patient who entrusts body and life to my judgment and sees me as their very own advocate. It is the sad truth that my judgments are reduced to second place under corporate profit as determined by a computer algorithm.

You must have an exact diagnosis in order to even have a computer code. How often is chronic fatigue an exact programmable condition? The world of health care is now offended by the intrusion of dollar driven non-health professionals, case reviewers, pharmaceutical denials, and limited time allotments for doctor care of patients. It is the death of trust between patient and doctor which I could no longer stomach. There was no compromise I could accept.

I practiced medicine for decades, feeling good about what I did. I cannot function when I need to receive permission before giving my patient what I deem necessary. I do not heal via recipe, or computer printout, no matter how "*expert*" the system. I needed room to allow thinking. I needed time to say hello and listen to what my patient did or did not say. The plague of denial in tests, treatments, prescriptives and such is as dangerous as The Black Plague.

There are physicians who can accept this. I could not. I could not make medical decisions, when 75 percent of the time, the decisions had to be influenced by capitation, insurance issues, and the judgment displayed not by science but by accounting, and I would be blamed for my denials. The "*innocent*" plan presents the doctor as the ultimate evil - by design.

Physicians and patients are being burned alive. The economic philosophy, terms of employment, and cash flow per share replace the human covenant of brotherhood between doctor and patient. Spirituality and the healing process have been fed to the furnaces.

I hear my friends telling me not to let myself get cynical. It's good advice. For awhile. But as the atrocities continue decade after decade, I begin to realize that we are all denying reality by being so determinedly upbeat in the face of the tragedy of the world. I'm sorry, but it is time to get a little cynical folks.

No, I have given up the practice of medicine for many reasons. My conscience demanded it. So did my nightly ability to fall asleep.

We must all note the price we pay for stupidity unchallenged, the price of selfishness, and the price of profit at any cost. George Bernard Shaw said, "*This is the true joy of life, the being used for a purpose recognized by yourself as a mighty one; the being thoroughly worn out before you are thrown on the scrap heap.*" To this I add, "*the being*" a force of nature instead of a feverish selfish clod of ailments and grievances complaining the world will not devote itself to making you happy, even as you destroy it.

Dr. Menninger remarked, "*Unrest of spirit is a mark of life. One problem after another presents itself, and in the solving of them, we find our greatest joys. The continuous encounter with continually changing conditions is the very substance of living. From an acute awareness of struggling effort, we have the periodic relief of seeing one task finished and another begun. A querulous search for a premature permanent peace seems to me a thinly disguised wish to die.*"

I do not believe our health is only a matter of machinery and muscle, blood and iron. We cannot be healthy without a morality, an ethic, which calls our conscience to order, and connects us to our fellow human beings. Let the healer's voice be heard!

We are asking for self affirmation, not just a bone marrow transplant, which we also demand when indicated. We cannot have health in any larger sense without social justice. Why do these words always scare us so? We must be heard!

We have compromised ourselves to death. We must re-invent the wheel if need be. We must re-invent idealism, optimism, and our dependence upon each other. We may be flawed, or lost and sick, but all of us have the capacity to be gloriously, triumphantly, proudly, human and therefore healing is within us.

Only a shared planet can survive. We need a new inspirational, ethical, scientific humanism. Medical researchers have been stymied too long. They must return to the support base of a government and university which cherishes academic research without imprisoning it. "*Die gedanken sind frei*" (Thought is free) in the words of the great old German university song. Why have we forgotten this?

Have we lost our wonder and surmise? If we modify our thoughts, and our behaviors, we can unlock peace. Is sanity and health only a beautiful dream of a tiny minority? It is our choice!

We have stared into the abyss for almost 100 years. Now we must move through, and past, our biases and our negativisms. We need to get rid of our rhetorical and theological ghosts. We must immediately dismiss the fear of eternal damnation! We need to move into a welcoming and peaceful future. Never doubt it!

There is something wrong with America when we have the largest prison population of any developed nation. We must no longer let the accidents of fate and irresponsibility turn our brothers and sisters into animals. We must find a way to keep the civil discourse civil. Notice that I am not saying we "*should*" do these things. I am saying that we "*must*" do these things! Do not despair.

The potentiality for greatness is everywhere. We can begin to lean away from death and toward education, toward community, toward the many (not just one!) statesmanlike politicians, even as the distance we must travel to reach our goal numbs our mind. If the American colonies could find 10 great men to form the United States of America, surely we, with 100 times as many people, can somehow find another 10 great men to lead us once again? Dear reader, I am talking about you and me! We can begin!

All of us are at disaster central, at ground zero. We're here, now, and the need is great. None of us know first hand anymore how irresistible a free people can be. We will find we are powerful. We will find our healing.

Yes your father murdered mine and mine murdered yours for 500 years, or 2500 years. We have all murdered and degraded each other, and the world is filled with our walking wounded and our bones. Our pain and our hate are almost unbearable! There will never be a moment when the scale is exactly equal. We will never be ready for peace. We will never be equal. We will never be healed!

That said, let us sit down together. Let us share our food, and talk. Let us leave our guns at the door, and laugh. In spite of everything, in spite of all the right on your side, in spite of all the violence on mine, and all the blood that lies between us, the time has come. No matter how ignorant we are, how prone to fury and red murder, the time has come at last. The time has come for peace. The time has come for health.

We can no longer expect the situation to somehow calm down and get better without intervention. The only time in our history remotely like today came during the breakup of the Roman Empire. We can't wait for another generation. The Empire is falling!

The New Age is dawning on a slippery slope. A Dark Age also beckons. The survivors could easily look back in hate from their straw hovels, 1000 years in the future. The future is in our hands. There is no more time!

A few men (they were almost all men) in Athens, between 450 and 400 B.C.E., created our civilization. What they did in the lifetime of one man has informed our world for 2400 years. Now we have finally reached the limits of what they first explored so long ago. Now, frighteningly, it is our turn to invent civilization!

We are on the edge! For one of the few times in human history, we are on the edge of a great leap into the unknown. Through all the Dark ages, for the last 1500 years, without realizing it, we had the security of retracing lost ground. We have haltingly re-created the civilizations of antiquity.

The job is now complete. Now what? Now we falter, in anger and fear and confusion, full of the tension of creation and expanded consciousness. We inevitably see our world as a falling apart, as chaos. It would be so easy to retreat into the consolations of the past.

It doesn't have to look that way. Let us use the best of our mind, our body, and our spirit, both to achieve wellness and happiness for ourselves, and to do our share to create the future. If we don't falter, we can build upon the loved ancient insights and come to a new insight, a new health, and a new world. Let us integrate our body, mind, and spirit and use the resulting wholeness to live. I welcome you with arms outstretched. Let us walk together.

When health, defined in the broadest sense, is so close, and the opportunity is so great, and the adventure beckons so frighteningly, we must not let the eternal presence of the Old Tempter take us back into chaos, superstition and Night. Forget Washington, D.C.! Our present rulers are bankrupt and totally irrelevant. Smug and self satisfied human beings never change.

**The Light beckons to those of us for whom the world shudders.**

Our great task is to create a new health and a new civilization, in a great act of synthesis and creation, for the entire human race, one person at a time! "*Whoever does not deserve a new world built in his or her time should consider it as being destroyed in his or her time.*" What a glorious opportunity!

The more clearly we are seen by the world, the more we are real. As I look into my dog's eyes, something looks back. The "*other*" (something outside the self) looks back at us all from earth and sky and sea. Fantasy and dream and imagination are precursors of consciousness. The registering brain of the crocodile sees us without dream. His eyes are sharp.

Only when we are conscious can we imagine consciousness. As we grow through life, becoming more and more conscious, we see more and more consciousness around us in the world. The entire earth is conscious to the holy ones.

Fantasy, dream, and imagination could fill our schools with light. Listen to me! **Fantasy, dream, and imagination could fill our schools with light!**

There is a quotation I have carried around in my wallet for 40 years:

*"Because everything we do and everything we are is in jeopardy, and because the peril is immediate and unremitting, every person is the right person to act and every moment is the right moment to begin, starting with the present moment."*

During the many years I was on the air talking about health I always felt an element of transcendence, something more than the ordinary, a hope for betterment for someone other than myself. It became almost automatic for me (it wasn't scripted) to sign off with, "*Take care of yourself, and each other. Till we meet again, good-bye and God bless.*" The funny thing is, I meant it.

The most important vitamin of all is vitamin L - for Love. I send you megadoses.

# THE END

www.ingramcontent.com/pod-product-compliance
Ingram Content Group UK Ltd.
Pitfield, Milton Keynes, MK11 3LW, UK
UKHW041948190726
13854UKWH00004B/1848

9 781552 123942